Praise for *Breaking the Fat Pattern*

"Excellent . . . [learn] how dieters ambush themselves . . . [as well as] many ideas for substitutions that save calories."

—*USA Today*

"Throw away those gimmicky diet books. To learn the secrets of managing your weight and health safely and effectively, this is the only one you will ever need. Highly recommended."

—John P. Foreyt, PhD, director of the Behavioral Medicine Research Center, Baylor College of Medicine in Houston, Texas

"In this refreshing guide to dropping pounds, readers learn how to assess their own bodies and whatever mental approaches they may have to dieting. Platkin['s] . . . approach is blessedly jargon-free and common-sense. Reading this book should help readers identify their negative eating patterns so that they can break them and replace them with healthier 'automatic' ones."

—*Publishers Weekly*

"It's about time! Amidst all the 'diet clutter,' here's a book—by an expert who's been in the trenches—that's sound in its science as well as simple and sensible."

—Hope S. Warshaw, MMSc, RD, author of *Guide to Healthy Restaurant Eating* and *Diabetes Meal Planning Made Easy*

"*Breaking the Fat Pattern* empowers the reader to formulate his/her own diet and exercise program that will work as effectively in the future as it does in the present."

—Dr. Howard M. Shapiro, *Picture Perfect Weight Loss*

Also by Charles Stuart Platkin

Breaking the Pattern: The Five Principles
You Need to Remodel Your Life

BREAKING
THE
FAT PATTERN

The Diet Detective's Plan
to End the Cycle of Yo-Yo Dieting

Charles Stuart Platkin

Previously published as *The Automatic Diet*

A PLUME BOOK

PLUME
Published by Penguin Group
Penguin Group (USA) Inc., 375 Hudson Street, New York, New York 10014, U.S.A.
Penguin Group (Canada), 90 Eglinton Avenue East, Suite 700, Toronto, Ontario, Canada M4P 2Y3
(a division of Pearson Penguin Canada Inc.)
Penguin Books Ltd., 80 Strand, London WC2R 0RL, England
Penguin Ireland, 25 St. Stephen's Green, Dublin 2, Ireland (a division of Penguin Books Ltd.)
Penguin Group (Australia), 250 Camberwell Road, Camberwell, Victoria 3124, Australia
(a division of Pearson Australia Group Pty. Ltd.)
Penguin Books India Pvt. Ltd., 11 Community Centre, Panchsheel Park, New Delhi – 110 017, India
Penguin Group (NZ), cnr Airborne and Rosedale Roads, Albany, Auckland 1310, New Zealand
(a division of Pearson New Zealand Ltd.)
Penguin Books (South Africa) (Pty.) Ltd., 24 Sturdee Avenue,
Rosebank, Johannesburg 2196, South Africa

Penguin Books Ltd., Registered Offices: 80 Strand, London WC2R 0RL, England

Published by Plume, a member of Penguin Group (USA) Inc. Previously published in a Hudson Street Press edition.

First Plume Printing, January 2006
10 9 8 7 6 5 4 3 2 1

The Library of Congress has catalogued the Hudson Street Press edition as follows:

Platkin, Charles Stuart.
    The automatic diet : the proven 10-step process for breaking your fat pattern / Charles Stuart Platkin.
        p. cm.
    Includes bibliographical references and index.
    ISBN 1-59463-000-3 (hc.)
    ISBN 0-452-28534-8 (pbk.)
    1. Weight loss. 2. Health behavior. I. Title.

RM222.2.P566 2005
613.2'5—dc22

2004054267

Printed in the United States of America

This book is dedicated to my daughter,
Parker South, a constant inspiration; to my
parents, Linda and Norton, who have always
and continue to be a driving force in my life;
and to my wife, a patient, considerate,
and caring friend, Shannon.

◄◄◄ ACKNOWLEDGMENTS ►►►

This book has been in the works for years, and I have many people to thank for helping me finally bring it to fruition.

First, I would like to thank my literary agent, Scott Waxman, a calm force in my turbulent, busy life—nothing seems to throw him off track. He believed in me from the start and has become a real friend.

Laureen Rowland, wow! What can I say—she is and will continue to be a powerhouse in publishing. I want to thank her for being a wonderful editor, and for pushing and challenging me to create a book that will make us both proud—and that reflects my true passion. I also want to thank her for understanding and believing in me as an author and as a person.

I would like to thank Judy Kern for her wit, commitment, calmness, confidence, and dedication (answering my phone calls, day or night by the second ring—seven days a week). But I owe her my gratitude mostly for her astounding patience (especially after the fifteenth change or addition to the manuscript after it was "completed") and her exceptional editorial capabilities.

Meredith Abreu, for her continued support, for being an uncompromising critic, and for her belief in me through thick and thin.

I would like to thank Richard Patton, RD, MPH, MS, who taught me how to apply the knowledge and scientific research to my thoughts and beliefs.

Shira Isenberg, RD, for those painstaking Wednesdays making sure the sentences worked and that what I wrote with passion made sense to everyone, not just me.

Carey Clifford, MS, RD, for listening to my ideas and acting as a sounding board in pursuit of changing people's lives.

Carole McCarthy, MSW, for helping to crystallize the behaviors necessary to help others help themselves.

Dr. Barbara J. Rolls, for taking the time out of her very busy life to be a continuous supporter of behavioral change and for her dedication to finding solutions to the obesity crisis.

Connie deSwaan, for helping me to get this book into a readable format, and for being a continuous ally.

◄◄◄ CONTENTS ►►►

◄◄◄ FOREWORD ►►►

Barbara Rolls, PhD

It is difficult to get through a day without hearing about America's epidemic of obesity. As we become more aware of the health problems associated with overweight and obesity, we are rushing to the bookstores to buy the latest, fad, diet book. Yet sensible people who, when faced with any other serious health problem would research the effectiveness of various treatments, often don't check out the science behind various weight-loss claims to determine if they are credible. I think a big part of why we keep searching for miraculous solutions to being overweight is that eating is such a fundamental and frequent part of who we are.

Surveys show that people fear that losing weight means giving up favorite foods forever. So we think in terms of quick fixes. We want to get the weight off as fast as we can and then get back to normal. If you think that way or if you have trouble maintaining the weight you have lost, then you should read *Breaking the Fat Pattern*. It will take you step-by-step through a process of self-analysis that will lead you to an understanding of your own patterns of success and failure in managing your weight. Charles Platkin will help you to get into your own head to understand the positive behaviors you can sustain and the self-defeating ones you need to shed.

Despite the dismal figures showing that most dieters regain their lost weight, we all know people who have broken this fat pattern. When I talk with such successes, it is clear that something changed in their heads. They had what Platkin describes as an "Aha" moment. Whether it was because of a health concern or a glimpse in the mirror, they suddenly got it—they had to take action. This book is going to show you how to have your own "Aha" moment. It will show you why you need to give up searching for a magic solution and focus instead on a personalized plan that systematically leads you to strategies that will help you sustain healthy eating and activity patterns and maintain weight loss automatically.

What is most impressive about this book is that it is serious about helping you to succeed in the long-term. Mr. Platkin himself struggled in the past with being overweight. Through his own personal experiences and those of the many people he has helped to manage their weight, he has developed a number of innovative, science-based tools to help people succeed at weight loss. You can tell from his writing that he has a personal interest in helping you to achieve long-term goals that will keep you fit and healthy.

He urges you to understand why quick fixes should be avoided. He then takes you on a personal voyage to help you discover what it takes to succeed with long-term weight management. You are encouraged to travel through a series of steps that systematically help you reveal the positive behaviors you are likely to make second nature and those that may defeat your best intentions. You are going to figure out why, despite your resolve, you ate that doughnut on the way to work. He does not blame you for such self-defeating behavior, but instead helps you understand what you are doing and why, and how to develop the motivation required to sustain more positive behaviors.

You will discover that the "secret" to long-term success is to have a personal strategy based on the positive behaviors that you can sustain. *Breaking the Fat Pattern* shows you how to evaluate your eating behavior and activity patterns to determine the healthful patterns that can become daily habits—like brushing your teeth. And, no, you will not be deciding between broccoli and chocolate. Platkin emphasizes that small changes in both diet and physical activity can add up to significant calorie savings. He directs you to healthy food choices and activities that can easily fit into the busiest day.

He has put together a personalized, inspirational, and practical guide to what the latest scientific advances tell us about weight management. So if you are serious about achieving a healthy weight and maintaining it, let Charles Platkin show you how to break the fat pattern.

Introduction

Let's get real about diets. Regardless of the diet du jour or the fact that you may have even lost a few pounds on it, old-fashioned, quick-weight-loss diets inevitably fail. Not only that, but after the diet's done, we gain back every precious pound we lost—and then some. But why does this have to happen?

It happens because, regardless of the gimmick or program, by their nature these diets prescribe a rigid eating plan that does not fit *anyone's* lifestyle over the long term. And they also fail because they often require a drastic reduction in calories that triggers the body's famine-survival mechanism, which slows down your metabolism. Instinctively, your body wants you to survive, while your stomach and thighs say, "I just want to lose a few pounds around the middle!"

So what *can* we do to lose weight and really keep it off?

The answer is not a better one-size-fits-all diet, but rather a clear understanding of what I call your individual fat pattern: how it works, and why you've been unable to lose and maintain your weight loss. *Breaking the Fat Pattern* is a step-by-step *process* that teaches you what to do so that you can take weight off—and keep it off. What it's *not* is another program for you to follow blindly so that you regain the weight you've lost six months after you've lost it. Rather, what you will learn is how to rethink the mechanisms that worked against you in the past so that they now work in your favor. By doing that, you will be able to develop new patterns of behavior to replace those that have failed in past. You will create an automatic, livable "diet" that works now—and in the future. And I'll be giving you proven methods for doing that, as well as practical strategies for implementing them so that they become second nature.

The process works by teaching you to become aware of the disappointing dieting patterns that have prevented you from achieving success—and to take responsibility for how those patterns affect the way you live.

I'm a big believer in expectation management, and I think you deserve to know, before you begin the process, what you're going to get out of it and why I'm the right person to help you end the cycle of dieting déjà vu.

I became a nutrition and public-health consumer advocate because I had discovered firsthand how maddening and futile quick-weight-loss diets were—high-protein, low-protein, low-fat, high-fat, grapefruit, no fruit—they all simply reduced calories by limiting the variety of foods I could eat. Highly restrictive and impossible to maintain over the long term, these diets all failed me and millions of others. I had been overweight my entire life, and I had given the responsibility for my weight loss to one fad diet after another. (In fact, in 1972, when I was just ten years old, I pleaded with my parents to buy me Dr. Atkins's diet book so that I could finally lose weight.) But once I understood and was able to apply the principles I'll be sharing with you in *Breaking the Fat Pattern*, I did an about-face and was able to lose more than fifty pounds—and, perhaps even more important, have kept it off for ten years.

It all began when I was a writing a book about how people can and can't change, and cynically thinking they couldn't, when, to my surprise, I discovered—after years of research and interviews on behavior modification, motivation, achievement, and personal responsibility—that a "leopard can actually change its spots." People *can* change. In fact, the science of behavioral change has a long and successful history. Its principles have allowed people to change their weight—and their lives. That first book, *Breaking the Pattern*, was a synthesis of what I'd discovered, and I'm proud to say that it has now been used by more than twenty universities around the country as a text for teaching behavioral change techniques to nutrition and dietetic counseling students.

Researching and writing *Breaking the Pattern* and my passion for public health subsequently led to my developing and writing one of the most widely syndicated weekly nutrition and fitness columns in the United States. The column now appears in more than 155 daily newspapers including the *Seattle Times,* the *New York Post,* the *Buffalo News,* the *Miami Herald,* the *Orange County Register,* the *Richmond Times-Dispatch,* and the *Honolulu Advertiser,* just to name a few.

I am also the founder and director of The Institute for Nutrition & Behavioral Sciences, a nonprofit organization that is currently conducting two studies, one focused on using the Internet as a means to counsel adolescents to help them lose weight (using a modified version of the process in this book), and the other a pilot, public-health program in southern Florida called Think Before You Eat, an educational campaign designed to create awareness about healthier eating by using a variety of media outlets.

In addition, two companies I founded are directly involved in delivering weight-control and health information and advice to individuals throughout the country.

iWellness Solutions is responsible for developing a sophisticated online technology-based software integrating cutting-edge scientific research and the latest in behavioral nutrition information, which is used by insurance companies, pharmaceutical companies, fitness centers, and large corporations, to assist more than 500,000 people each year in losing weight and increasing their physical activity.

Nutricise is the first program to provide individuals one-on-one weight-control counseling with registered dietitians via email. Nutricise is based on the principles of behavioral nutrition, and has now counseled more than 65,000 people, helping them to understand that choosing to lose weight is not simply about choosing what we put in our mouths, it's about choosing how we live our lives.

My proven methods have been refined and simplified to include only what actually works, and Nutricise has been given high marks by *Fitness* magazine (which recognized it as the "only program of its kind that offers such intensely personalized counseling"), *PC Magazine,* and *Newsweek* as one of the best interactive diets available. Additionally, *Men's Health* sent an undercover registered dietitian to try out the various diet programs available online, and the Nutricise program came out on top, the only site to receive four-out-of-four stars. The site has also been voted *Forbes* magazine's "Favorite" and "Best of the Web," as well as one of *Health* magazine's "Top 25 Web Sites for Women."

Now, I want to share those same techniques with you.

* * *

The theories and techniques in *Breaking the Fat Pattern* are based on authoritative, scientific studies, which have repeatedly shown that quick-fix diets are misguided and ultimately useless because they focus on advocating or restricting particular foods when the only really effective way to lose and maintain weight loss over time is by carefully reviewing one's past diet history, learning key behavioral strategies, and making small but significant alterations in one's eating and physical activity. What this book will teach you is exactly how to do that.

Most diets tell you that to lose weight you have to change your life, alter everything you've been doing, and follow *their* prescription. Everything is done for you by the program. And, as a result, you lose touch with the most important part of losing weight, which is having the ability to manage your own biological and psychological needs.

Learning to do that is not difficult once you accept the core concept that any maintainable weight-control program must be based on *compromise, not conformity.* What this means is that you need to compromise with yourself, not conform to someone else's definition of who you *should* be. If you conform, you're following someone else's diet—a prescription that might sound great on paper and that may work in the short run. To succeed in the long run, however, you need to find your own perfect fit, a way of eating and living that's been custom-made for you—not something that's been pulled off the "ready-to-wear" diet rack—and you do that by compromising with the one person who really matters: *you!*

To this you may respond, "I *want* someone else to tell me what to do and eat—figuring it out for myself sounds too hard!" But it's not. To teach you how, I'll provide you with the simple tools and straightforward strategies you need to become a successful "diet detective," understand your unique fat patterns, identify "Calorie Bargains," and come up with a livable diet that works for a lifetime.

Like any learning process, this one begins with the basics. Then, after taking a few simple steps, you'll move on to the next level, until, at the end of your 10-step process you'll be an expert on the subject of your own personal weight management.

In Part 1, Compromise, Don't Conform, you'll first come to understand that all standardized diets fail in the long term because they ask us to conform to someone else's plan when what we really need to do is discover why we've failed in the past (our personal fat pattern) and determine how we can compromise with *ourselves* in order to change those patterns and live with the changes for the rest of our lives.

Once you understand that, you can begin to create a livable diet by looking for Calorie Bargains and making the small changes in eating behavior that will put you on the path toward permanent weight loss. You'll also learn how to create a personal food environment and automate the behaviors that will help to ensure your success.

Then, to ensure that you don't stray from the path you need to be on to reach your goal, I'll be teaching you how to do the investigative detective work that will allow you to bring your past fat patterns out into the open by looking at your Individual Dieting Traits (IDTs), and then giving you practical advice *you can use right now* to cope with Unconscious Eating, your Eating Alarm Times, and those Diet Buster situations and occasions when you're most likely to fall off your diet.

At that point, it will be time to add the next necessary component of change—increasing your activity level so that you'll be burning calories faster. You'll learn new ways of doing that without subjecting yourself to hours of running, rigorous weight training, or getting in shape for the next triathlon. Again, the changes I'll be asking you to make are small but significant. And you'll be finding the ones that will work with your life, not committing to those that require you to change your life altogether.

Armed with those basics, it will be time to move on to Part 2: Empower, Not Willpower.

Willpower, as I learned for myself and I'm sure you've already discovered, simply isn't tough enough to overcome temptation every time. With that in mind, I'll be providing you with strategies that will empower you to use the tools you've already acquired without having to depend on the fickle frailty of willpower alone.

First, you'll learn what it takes to stop sabotaging yourself by playing the Blame Game (shifting the responsibility for your failures onto situations or circumstances you believe are beyond your control) and find out how to use Excuse Busters to neutralize the very human tendency to talk yourself out of doing what you know you should.

Then, to help you use that control, I'll explain the power of skillful long- and short-term planning to achieve your weight-loss goals, and I'll teach you how to Think—and Make It Happen by using visualization to create an imagined, meaningful, detailed vision of your life *after* you've reached your goal weight that will help you keep the faith in the midst of hard food choices. You'll also learn how Mental Rehearsal can allow you to practice how you will behave in difficult situations so that when they occur, you'll be able to make the choices that will support the changes you're creating. And finally, you'll be using everything you've learned to create your own, personal, blueprint for success.

Again, my goal is not to preach, not to give complicated, unrealistic, "cheerleader" advice, or a prescription that will fail over time, but instead to provide practical, simple, and concise steps to help you take control of your weight by recognizing, breaking, and replacing the patterns that have led to your being overweight.

Ten steps in all, each one building on the other. The process is designed to be tasty and comfortable so that it should feel like a walk in the park, but that doesn't mean it will be easy and require no effort. Like any walk with a specific destination, however, if you just keep putting one foot in front of the other, you *will reach your goal*—and that's a guarantee.

We are all, principally, the authors of our own lives, and we have the power, in spite of genetics, environment, and/or our slow metabolisms, to write a different outcome than the one we see on the scale each day. You are now at the beginning of the end of dieting déjà vu.

▶▶▶▶▶▶▶▶▶▶▶▶▶▶▶▶▶▶▶▶▶▶ **PART I**

Compromise,
Don't Conform

What is it that's preventing you from reaching your weight-loss goal? Is it your slow metabolism? Stressful job? An underactive thyroid? Unsupportive spouse? Fluctuating hormones? No time or money to do what you think you need to do to lose the weight? Is this just not the right point in your life to start focusing on a *diet*? Are you genetically predisposed to being overweight, just like your parents?

Well, it's time to come to grips with the fact that a mega-dose of willpower is not going to appear in your breakfast cereal tomorrow morning. Cursing the fates is not going to change your hormones, genetics, or metabolism, and the next quick-fix diet you go on is not going to be *the one that does it—the* "diet" that finally defeats all your obstacles to losing weight for life.

So, what is it then? What *will* help you lose weight forever? What is the "Big Secret"? Well, after years of research as a nutrition, fitness, and weight-loss consumer advocate; as a public health lecturer with a master's degree in public health and nutrition, and the founder of a successful health, nutrition, and weight control company; as a certified personal trainer; and as someone who has counseled tens of thousands of clients and personally lost fifty pounds (keeping it off for more than ten years), I have the answer:

> *You can't simply go on a "diet" and make the fat disappear forever. But you* **can** *change how you think about dieting and fat, and that* **will** *make the fat disappear forever!*

Before I shed the weight myself, and learned the techniques that worked, I went on any and every diet as far back as I can remember. I've probably been on diets you've never even heard of, and each of my dieting experiences ended in dismal failure. Oh, don't get me wrong—all the diets worked, for a while. I *did* lose weight. But one of the key questions about weight loss I needed to have answered is what happens *after* you lose those ten, twenty, or even one hundred pounds? You probably already know—you gain the weight back.

The fact is, most people come to a diet to drop flab fast, and if the diet helps them to do that, they don't much care how or why it works. But if the objective of a diet plan is to help you lose weight and *keep it off,* you must learn how to *adjust your behavior for a lifetime, not just for a few weeks.* Now, I'm not saying that you have to revamp your whole life all at once, or that you have to stop eating everything you love. *What I am saying is that you need to create a program that is livable and automatic, and as you read through this book, I will teach you how to adjust what you are doing now so that you can, in effect,* automatically *lose and maintain weight loss in your future.*

Once I've given you those tools and strategies, you'll have the knowledge and the power to do the rest yourself. The diets that haven't worked for you before promise to do the work for you; They say if you live by *their* rules, you will be successful. By now, however, you've realized that living by their rules doesn't work. What does work, as you'll come to understand, is empowering yourself to make small changes and compromises with yourself, so that you can live with your new, slimmer self for the rest of your life.

This is what most diet and weight-loss experts tell you to do:

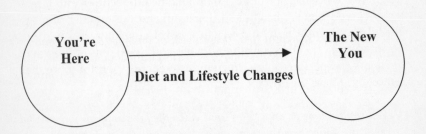

This is what you should be doing:

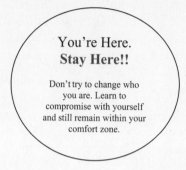

You're Here.
Stay Here!!

Don't try to change who
you are. Learn to
compromise with yourself
and still remain within your
comfort zone.

Before you can even begin to do that, however, you need to make one very important decision. You need to choose.

Making the Choice

The bottom line is that you have two choices:

Choice 1: You can choose to accept responsibility for your weight, deal with the obstacles and challenges you face, and make up your mind to lose the weight. No matter what your problem, situation, or circumstance, the solution is still the same: You're the one who is responsible, and losing weight has to be what *you* really want. In fact, a study reported in the *International Journal of Obesity and Related Metabolic Disorders* has found that those people who believe their weight problems result from choices they have made rather than from metabolism or genetics were more successful at losing weight because they believed they were *in control* of their weight loss. *Does this mean you have to be superhuman?* Not at all—it simply means that you need to want something, take it seriously, and take the time in the beginning to set yourself up with the tools you need to make it happen. With this attitude and emotionally charged choice, this book will help you get to your desired weight—and stay there.

OR

Choice 2: You can choose to remain overweight. And, harsh as this may sound, make no mistake: If you continue to be overweight, it is something *you* have *chosen*.

Let's assume you've made choice number one. If so, I can promise you that whether you've picked up *Breaking the Fat Pattern* as a companion to a diet you're already on, to help you lose weight after you've been on another diet, or to maintain a recent weight loss, you will walk away from reading this book with a new understanding and a set of skills that are based on the latest scientific research and that have worked for me and thousands of my clients.

As you begin to practice these new skills, I can promise that they will become automatic. You will no longer have to think about them because they will be working, on a subconscious level, to keep you trim and healthy forever.

◀◀◀ STEP 1 ▶▶▶

Accept the Truth About Diets

"Believe nothing, no matter where you read it, or who said it, no matter if I said it, unless it agrees with your own reason and your common sense."
—Buddha

"Bring your stretch pants."
—Advertisement for Roadhouse Grill All-You-Can-Eat Program

The first step toward breaking your fat pattern is to understand why all those diets you've already been on both do and don't work. Having the complete picture will guide you through and keep you focused on making lasting change because insight into why you are doing something is sometimes as important as doing it. In this first Step, you will learn about your body's ancient survival mechanism, the role genetics really does play in the weight-loss game, how powerful your personal environment can be in reducing your waistline, and, finally, how success can become automatic. Believe me, there's nothing written in stone—or in your genes—that you don't have the power to change.

Do You Believe in Miracles?

Too many of us are perplexed (and frustrated for that matter) when it comes to dieting and weight loss. There are many good reasons for the confusion. Every day we are inundated with "miracle" products that promise to solve our weight-loss problems: The latest quick-fix diet books lead the bestseller lists. Manufacturers market special drinks, and diet supplements promise a better body in weeks. Television commercials showcase gimmicks promising to burn calories without our moving a muscle and feature testimonials from people who have lost tremendous amounts of weight on one program or another. All of this media exposure adds up to a $50 billion weight-loss industry—yet, as a nation, we get fatter and fatter every year.

We buy low-calorie, low-carb, and low-fat products, deny ourselves delicious foods, drink only artificially sweetened soda, buy specially prepared meals and drinks, join fitness centers, take diet pills, submit to liposuction or gastric-bypass surgery, and, when we're feeling especially motivated, work out obsessively to burn off calories.

I can tell you from firsthand experience, despite what the products and advertisements claim, there's no magic formula or quick-fix solution for permanent weight loss. (And unfortunately, I haven't read any research that indicates a "miracle" will be coming anytime soon.) So don't expect this book to provide a "quick-and-easy" healthy recipe for success to which you just add water and artificial sweetener, then stir. *If you think something will jump off the pages of this book and lose the weight for you without your own committed input, don't walk, but run (even though it might involve some exercise) back to the bookstore and get your money back.* If there were one simple specific answer to everyone's diet dilemmas, you'd have heard about it by now, and almost 70 percent of Americans wouldn't be overweight.

But what this book *can* give you are the essential ingredients and strategies you need to identify your own *fat patterns*—those unique circumstances, situations, and behaviors (including eating and physical activity) that have led to your own particular weight problem. With these tools you will be able to break those negative patterns and create a life that does not have to focus obsessively on dieting and losing weight because doing what's necessary will become automatic.

The Diet of the Day

Most, if not all of us have fallen for the allure of a "quick-fix" diet at one time or another. How many times have *you* made that decision to finally lose the weight and get in shape? You're all excited. You promise yourself this is it—the *last time.* You pick the diet du jour, and you do it. You starve, suffer, and sacrifice—you make it happen. You have willpower—you're strong. The needle on the scale is moving toward the lower digits, so everything else is acceptable. As long as the pounds are dropping off, you can endure the suffering. The hope is that this time you'll lose the weight and it will all be over—you will never have to diet again.

Unfortunately, the quick-fix diet is like a dream lover—the hero or heroine who suddenly appears in our lives and promises to meet all our needs and solve all our problems. But, like the reality of the dream lover, the romance of the dream *diet* is just as elusive and disappointing. At some point, we're bound to wake up to the fact that we've fallen off our plan, that our hopes have not come true, and we're back where we started. Overweight.

So why do we do it to ourselves? Because, for a while, these diets do actually work—dieting and overhauling your entire life does help you to lose weight. In fact, the National Weight Control Registry—which tracks people who, on average, have successfully lost at least sixty pounds and maintained the loss for at least five years—has demonstrated that successful weight losers use a *variety* of dieting methods to shed their pounds. But if any number of diets will help you lose weight, why not simply pick any one on the market and just go for it?

Because the trick is that most of these diets are *designed* to work primarily in the short term. And I don't know about you, but I'd prefer *not* to gain weight back after I've lost it.

That's not to say, however, that there's nothing to be learned from these diets. And, in fact, if you've made the choice to be serious about ending your "fat" pattern, it's critical for you to understand why they do and don't work, what it is you *can* learn from them, and how to use "dieting" to your advantage. You need to know it all if you're going to succeed. So each time you read something that tempts you to say, "yes, but . . ." just be patient. Hang on to those great questions. I promise that the answers will be there for you in the pages of this book.

First of all, you should know that it is a generally accepted principle in the diet industry that the amount of weight you lose in the first four weeks of any diet will determine whether you continue on the program or move on. A significant initial weight loss, in other words, can be a powerful motivation for continuing. In fact, if you don't lose enough weight in those first four weeks—it's on to another diet. But ironically (and sadly), according to the *Journal of Consulting and Clinical Psychology*, one predictor of your potential to *regain* weight is how fast you lose it— meaning, the faster you lose the weight, the more likely you will be to gain it back.

So, you need to be aware that, whatever your initial success, none of these diets was *intended* to work in the long term. If you don't keep that in mind, you'll be getting sucked back into the fast, simple, easy, diet solutions that give you a quick fix and get you caught in the vicious cycle of dieting déjà vu.

Another major problem with quick-weight-loss diets is that when you lose weight on some of them, you're not only losing fat; many times you're losing water and lean muscle mass. And when people lose muscle, their metabolism slows down. Muscle mass is the body's most efficient furnace. The more muscle you have, the more calories your body burns, whether you're sitting reading a book or working out in the gym, so the more muscle you lose, the harder it will become to lose weight. But does that mean every quick diet is going to cause you to lose muscle mass and water? And why would anyone continue on these types of diets given all the negative consequences, especially with their dismal success rates?

Because, in the end, diets can be both good and bad, and some are healthier than others. The healthier ones don't involve quick weight loss as one of their components (on a healthy diet you should lose about ½ pound to 2 pounds per week), they generally help you make good food choices, and they put you on track. So you need to understand what a quickie diet will and will not do for you. You need to be an educated consumer.

You can learn from all of them, and once you've learned what works for you, you can apply what's worked in the past to what you'll be doing in the future. If you don't, you'll just keep on doing what you've been doing, and you know what the outcome of that will be; you've been there before.

The main reason for understanding how and why diets work is that the more you know about them the better chance you'll have of achieving weight-loss success, which is really what matters.

Why Diets Work: It's Simpler Than You Think

All crash diets begin with a claim as to why the plan works: more protein, less protein, all the bacon you want, all the cabbage you want, more fruit, no fruit, only fruit before noon—whatever. But the real secret behind all these diets is not the special combinations of foods or the magical qualities of one particular food, or even the right food for your body type: The "secret" is simply the restriction of food. That's right! Diets work because you're consuming fewer calories than you burn and your body is in a caloric deficit. It's cutting calories, and perhaps an increase in physical activity, that always results in weight loss. And that goes for all diets, including all the biggies: Atkins, South Beach, The Zone, Weight Watchers, Jenny Craig, even Dr. Phil's plan—they're all about the calories.

Calories by the Numbers

It's a fact that 3,500 calories makes up a pound. If your body needs 2,000 calories per day to function and maintain your weight, and you eat 2,500 calories per day, that's an additional 500 calories per day. That makes an additional 3,500 calories per week—which equals an extra pound gained.

Are there ways to make yourself *less* hungry with what and how you eat? Absolutely. That's what Atkins, South Beach, and other prescriptive programs attempt to create—a feeling of satisfaction during the initial stages of the diet so you feel more comfortable and don't suffer. Again, there are things we can learn from different diets.

Unfortunately, the reality is that it's impossible to lose as much weight as most quick-loss diets promise. For instance, even if we went on a total fast, it's unlikely that we would lose fifteen pounds in one week, as some of the more unrealistic diets claim we will. Take a look: If we deprived ourselves of every single one of our average 2,500 calories per day and multiplied that by seven days, it would equal 17,500 calories lost, or about five pounds. And that doesn't account for the slowing of our metabolism and loss of valuable water and lean muscle, which occur when we starve ourselves. The minute we replaced the water we'd have lost, we would regain some of the weight. Then, most likely, we would binge on all the foods we were restricting, bringing on even more weight.

Or, let's do the math another way. To lose one pound of fat, you must burn 3,500 more calories than you eat. Say, for example, you weigh 170 pounds and are moderately active. Your calorie needs for weight maintenance are about 2,500 a day. If your diet contains only 1,500 calories, you'd have an energy deficit of 1,000 calories a day. In a week's time that would add up to a 7,000-calorie deficit, or only two pounds lost. Even in ten days, the accumulated deficit would represent only about three pounds of lost body fat.

But even if you *ate nothing at all for ten days* and maintained your usual level of activity, your caloric deficit would add up to 25,000 calories (2,500 calories a day times ten). At 3,500 calories per pound of fat, that's still only seven pounds of lost fat. So if you want to lose fat—not valuable water or muscle—the loss must be gradual, ranging from one to two pounds per week, or 1 to 2 percent of your total body weight.

Fat, Protein, Carbohydrates—Does It Matter?

Carefully controlled metabolic studies show that it doesn't matter where extra calories come from. Eat more calories than you expend and you'll gain weight, plain and simple.

I'm not saying that certain foods don't cause you to be hungrier sooner or that some foods don't digest more quickly while others help to keep your belly full longer. In fact, I'll be discussing just how that works when I give you the secrets of creating an automated, comfortable, eating and physical activity routine in Steps 2, 3, and 6.

For now, let's just say that it's one of the reasons why the Atkins, high-protein, high-fat diet is so popular—it helps you restrict calories without making you feel hungry or deprived.

Changing Your Breakfast

Let's say, for example, you *normally* eat two eggs scrambled with a tablespoon of butter, four slices of bacon, and two slices of rye toast with two tablespoons of butter for breakfast. This is what it would look like:

Two large eggs = 162 calories
Four slices of bacon = 100 calories
Three tablespoons of butter (one for the eggs, two for the toast)
= 300 calories

Two slices rye toast = 160 calories (approximately)
Total: 722 calories

Now, if you change to a high-protein, high-fat diet, you're eliminating the toast and the butter. As a result, you save 362 calories. Even if you added an extra egg, you'd still be saving 279 calories. Add an extra slice of bacon with the egg, and you'd still be saving 254 calories. And if you eliminated nothing more than those 254 calories, you'd be saving 1,778 calories every seven days and, without changing *anything else,* you'd lose a pound in less than three weeks.

So, once again, *it's those calories saved*, not the specific nutritional composition of the calories, that causes you to lose weight.

That doesn't mean, however, that a high-protein diet is necessarily "better" in long-term effectiveness than other diets. In fact, Dr. Gary Foster's groundbreaking research on low-carbohydrate diets, reported in the *New England Journal of Medicine,* showed that after one year, those who followed a low-carb diet hadn't lost any more weight than those who had followed the more conventional, high-carbohydrate, low-calorie approach.

Why Diets Don't Work

Why do our bodies resist diets? By definition, the word "diet" is a noun (not a verb) meaning "food and drink regularly provided or consumed," so how can you fail at something as easy as that? The problem is that we have given the word "diet" a negative spin. We have made it a term that conjures up neon lights that flash: RESTRICTION!, DON'T EAT!, BLAND!, NO TASTE!, and the list goes on.

The Starvation Trap

When we go on a diet—a euphemism for a degree of starvation—the body's ancient, survival mechanisms kick in, lowering our metabolic rate and thereby decreasing our energy as well as our energy requirements. The body doesn't know if it's starving itself voluntarily (to lose weight) or involuntarily (because there isn't any food available). And, since we're all genetically programmed with a fixed biological drive to survive, your body doesn't want your diet to succeed. Instead, it responds as if it's being starved rather than transformed into a "slim, new you." As Michael Lowe, PhD, a professor of psychology at Drexel University reported in *Obesity Research*, the body defends its weight defiantly, lowering its metabolism and refusing to use up valuable stored energy, thus making it more difficult to burn calories. And this effect is intensified by the mind's insistence on demanding food. The more you diet, the more you try not to eat, the stronger your mind and body defend their desire to eat. That doesn't mean you can't successfully and comfortably eliminate Ben & Jerry's from your nighttime routine. It simply means that your *desire* for Ben & Jerry's is not going to disappear.

Long before we had supermarkets and easy access to highly palatable food on virtually every corner, we humans were hunters and gatherers. It was either "feast" or "famine," so the body had to be prepared for both situations. The more we ate, the fatter we got, and the fatter we got, the better off we were when times of "famine" occurred, because each excess pound of fat provided us with additional days of life. Fat was, therefore, a valuable asset, as much as it's now become an albatross around our modern waists.

While we have evolved in many ways since those early times, our body's ability to regulate weight is still a few thousand years behind. For most of us, there is no longer a need to store fat in order to survive times of famine, but our bodies don't know that. The body still acts as if it's saving our life and continues to slow down in response to our depriving it of fuel. When we eat more, our metabolism speeds up; eat less, and it goes into "starvation mode," slowing down to compensate for the lack of calories. And, in addition, there is some evidence that the body, in its effort to become a fuel-efficient machine, also attempts to minimize our activity level by making us feel tired and lethargic, which, of course, means it will be even harder to burn calories. Not exactly what you want to happen when you're trying to lose weight.

Thus, the typical yo-yo dieting cycle emerges: The more effort you put into limiting your calories, the more your body resists weight loss. The numbers on the scale take a nosedive the first few weeks, and then the pounds stop coming off because your metabolism has slowed down. You become discouraged and disappointed; you "go off" your diet, and the weight comes right back, sometimes faster than you lost it, leaving you heavier than you were when you started.

It's True, Genes Do Count

Ever wonder why you seem to get hungry faster than a friend, even after consuming the same meal? Or why you're more likely than others to gain weight eating the same food as your best friend or spouse?

In his book, *What You Can Change and What You Can't,* researcher Dr. Martin Seligman makes a compelling case for the role genes play in weight management. "Nineteen out of twenty studies," he writes, "show that obese people consume no more calories each day than nonobese people. In one remarkable experiment, a group of very obese people dieted down to the point where they were 60 percent overweight and stayed there. But even to remain at 60 percent overweight, they had to consume one hundred *fewer* calories a day than normal people could consume to stay at normal weight."

Dr. Jules Hirsch of Rockefeller University, one of the foremost authorities and researchers on obesity, has also completed a variety of studies indicating that people who are overweight have a different genetic makeup from people of normal weight, and that being overweight is not always the result of being lazy or lacking in willpower. Instead, he argues, something programs obese individuals to store more fat than normal-weight people.

In fact, scientists have long known there is a significant genetic component to weight. Dr. James Levine, MD, PhD, reporting in *Science,* has demonstrated in his research that two people of the same gender, weight, age, and lifestyle, both of whom eat exactly the same number of calories each and every day, can, at the end of a year, have arrived at completely different weights. And it has also been shown that adopted children do not resemble the weights of their adoptive parents, but do resemble the weights of their natural parents.

While there is certainly evidence to indicate that some people will be genetically inclined to have a faster metabolism than others—burning more calories—it doesn't mean that those of us who are programmed to survive in times of famine need to feel hopeless because food is now plentiful. It does, however, indicate, as I've been saying all along, that there is no quick fix that's going to work for everyone. In fact, since we're all obviously so different, this book is exactly what you need to help you identify and reset your own negative patterns in a way no general diet plan can.

Maureen McGurie, PhD, reporting in *Obesity Research* concluded that maintaining weight loss is not impossible even for those who were overweight, but that it requires an attentive program tailored specifically to the individual that uses "more behavioral strategies" to help control weight. That doesn't mean, however, that your "attentiveness" needs to be all-consuming. The techniques in this book, which are based on compromise and geared to your individual lifestyle have been designed to provide you with strategies you can live with forever, new ways of thinking and behaving that will allow you—no matter what your genetic makeup, weight, or previous diet failures—to achieve your weight-loss goal and maintain what you've achieved forever. And, as you are about to learn, whatever your genetic makeup, *your environment, which is well within your control, is the factor that makes all the difference.*

Environment Counts, Too

Compelling evidence that genetics alone do not determine whether or not we will be overweight is supplied by a study done by the National Institutes of Health (NIH) on two tribes of Pima Indians.

Some years ago, a team of NIH researchers went to Sacton, Arizona, to study rheumatoid arthritis among the Pima who lived there. In the course of their investigations, the researchers uncovered another critical health issue in the tribe: The Pimas' diabetes rate was at 50 percent, eight times higher than the national average. And the Pimas were also *significantly overweight and obese*—in fact, they are one of the most obese ethnic groups in the world.

Meanwhile, another team of researchers studied a tribe of Mexican Pima Indians, performing the same tests as those done on the Arizona Pimas. Their studies found that the Mexican Pimas actually consumed *more* calories than their American counterparts. They were, however, far more physically active as well as comparatively thin, and the prevalence and incidence of diabetes was comparatively normal.

So even though both groups of Pima Indians have a similar genetic background, they have different disease rates *due to their respective environments and how they live.* This demonstrates that genetic makeup *can* be influenced by environment and your set point *can* be altered by lifestyle. As public health advocate Pamela Peeke, MD, MPH, put it, "Genetics may load the gun, but environment pulls the trigger."

Forbidden Cravings and Other Mental Stumbling Blocks

In addition to the biological stumbling blocks that are genetic and metabolic, there's an important psychological component to the failure of quick-weight-loss diets. If "diet" is simply another word for deprivation, it makes sense that any time we deny ourselves food we will want to eat more than ever. We tend to want things we can't have, so why would we think food was any different?

Because of this craving for the forbidden, our ability to lose weight through deprivation can be limited, which is yet another reason—in addition to preventing your body from thinking it's starving—for losing weight *gradually* by compromising rather than conforming. By doing that, you'll be able to keep those cravings under control.

I call these cravings, along with the other psychological factors we've already discussed, a "Diet Ambush."

Diet Ambush

Post-Deprivation Elation: As soon as the diet is over, the first thing post-dieters may do is gorge on all the foods (good and bad) the diet made off limits. They believe the diet has protected them against weight gain and that they can eat anything.

Diet-Failure Despair: If you've been on a diet and haven't lost as much weight as you'd wanted to, you'll be demoralized and won't even have the desire to try again.

The Energy Zap: Diets are exhausting. They take time, effort, and often don't provide enough calories for sustained energy.

The Craving Crazies: In addition to a slowed metabolism, deprivation creates exaggerated cravings, and so a piece of chocolate seems a million times more desirable than it really is. When people are on a diet, they tend to focus on deprivation, incessantly thinking about the foods they can't have. Of course, they become obsessed and respond with diet-induced overeating. And they never focus on what really matters—changing their behavior and how they think about food in relation to themselves.

So What Does All This Mean?

As we have seen, and scientists have long known, weight gain and obesity are the result of a multitude of genetic, biological, environmental, and psychological factors. But by reviewing, understanding, and learning to control how we react to these perceived obstacles, including a genetic predisposition to obesity, we *can* succeed in losing weight and keeping it off. In other words, controlling your weight really means learning to control the availability, composition, and portion size of the food in your personal environment, and monitoring your psychosocial behaviors with regard to food so that you will be able to intervene and modify those behaviors in real-world situations.

One British study, published in *Obesity Research,* stated the problem (and the solution) this way:

> Food intake (eating) is a form of behavior that is subject to conscious control. In practice, many obese and weight-gaining individuals claim that their eating is out of (their) control. Mechanistic models describe the interplay of biological and environmental forces that control food intake. However, because human food intake is characterized by individuals intervening to adjust their own patterns of behavior, food intake should reflect interactions among biology, environment, and *attempted self-imposed control of behavior.* [emphasis added]

If you think having confidence in yourself might not be particularly important for losing weight forever—think again. A study, conducted by Jacinda B. Roach, PhD, RD, and colleagues, and published in the *Journal of the American Dietetic Association* reports that when various methods for increasing confidence in their ability to control their weight and create their own outcome (e.g., reading empowering books, reviewing family history, nutrition education, and identifying their reasons for wanting to lose weight) participants' eating habits improved and their weight loss was greater.

The process I'll be taking you through in this book is designed to give you the kind of self-knowledge and skills that will evoke that very same confidence you need to make it happen.

To begin with, it ought to be obvious that once you lose weight, you need to keep the weight off by eating the same types of foods that helped shed the pounds—not by going back to consuming whole boxes of cookies in front of the TV. But it was never obvious to me. And, apparently, I'm not the only one who thought I'd become a member of the "eat-whatever-you-want" club.

I really believed that something had changed and that I wouldn't have to worry any more. That was my dream, but I now understand and accept that my dream simply needed to be altered slightly. I have found a place where I'm comfortable and happy—and able to control my weight—and so can you.

Join the 2% Club

Does this sound familiar: After losing those pounds you suddenly feel that, *overnight*, your body has changed, making you a charter member of the exclusive fast-metabolism-I-can-eat-whatever-I want club. For a few weeks in your new, fit body you are confident that the weight is off for good. You indulge—and the diet you had been on is now ancient history—because all along *you knew* you could never live on that diet for the rest of your life. In fact, according to the latest research published in the *International Journal of Obesity and Related Metabolic Disorders* and the *Annals of Internal Medicine*, almost everyone, about 98 percent of those who diet, will regain all the weight they lose within three to five years.

Then one morning you wake up, and the reflection in the mirror reveals a truth that cannot be denied. *You were NEVER in the club.* Not only have you regained the weight you lost, you've actually added *more pounds*. When this happens, you probably feel frustrated, ashamed, powerless, and you're probably ready to throw up your hands in defeat. And all that is okay, we've all felt that way at times, but the information in this book will give you the tools, encouragement, and power to move forward even after your most devastating defeat, so that you can become one of the 2 percent who keep the weight off forever!

If you use the strategies I outline to set yourself up to succeed and then make the small adjustments I suggest, I promise you that losing weight and keeping it off will become easier and easier, until it is virtually automatic. As Rena Wing, PhD, at Brown University School of Medicine reported in a landmark study: *Weight maintenance does get easier over time.*

It's As Simple As Brushing Your Teeth

If I told you that if you didn't brush your teeth every day you would end up toothless in a matter of years, and that you would have bad breath along with other vanity and health issues, what would you do? Would you stop brushing? Well, that wouldn't make any sense, right? Even though you believed that brushing your teeth was a chore, you'd see the value of doing it, so you would merely make the process part of your everyday life.

Well, overeating and not exercising have real consequences, just like not brushing your teeth. And, in fact, those consequences are significantly more serious (including heart disease, diabetes, cancer, depression, and decreased job opportunities) than chronic bad breath and a gummy grin. So, just like brushing your teeth, weight control needs to become part of your life—part of your daily routine—for it to be effective. Think of it along the same lines as showering, going to work, and taking care of your family. Sure, they're responsibilities, but they're manageable, and can even be enjoyable.

And keep this in mind—even if all the negative weight-loss research were conclusive (which it's not), it wouldn't matter because, with the efficient, empowering lifestyle agenda I'll be providing, you *can* change your weight. I know, because I did it—and believe me, I have very little innate willpower.

This Is for the Rest of Your Life

The key is to understand and accept that *making small lifestyle changes can have a significant impact on permanent weight loss.* Doing that will require *auditing your behaviors and making small changes you can live with for the rest of your life*—NOT overhauling your entire life, depriving yourself, making commitments to yourself that you can never keep, and then feeling badly about it (and yourself!).

It's important to develop your own, unique method of reducing and burning calories. Your plan needs to allow for individual differences and tastes and yet remain effective and easy to make an automatic part of your day—*each and every day*. Therefore, the one most important question you need to ask yourself before each and every small change is: *"Can I maintain this eating lifestyle forever?"*

Once you've answered "yes" to that question and determined to make the change, you will have *set a goal for yourself*. The next step is to determine when, where, and how you will implement that goal. Peter Gollwitzer, professor of psychology at New York University, calls this step "implementation intention," which he describes as linking "anticipated opportunities with goal-directed responses," or, with relation to your weight-loss goal, having decided in advance how you will *change your behavior* to *respond differently* to a potentially diet busting circumstance that has derailed you in the past.

In the following pages, I'll be showing you how important it is to rehearse and anticipate these circumstances so that they *don't* undermine your goals. And I'll be providing the simple strategies that have helped others not only to achieve their weight-loss goals, but also to succeed in every aspect of life, including business situations, personal relationships, and competitive sports.

It Will Become Automatic

As you'll be learning, the more you practice and implement these strategies, the more they will become a part of your everyday life, so that, before too long, they will be *automatic*. John Bargh and Tanya Chartrand, both members of the department of psychology at New York University at the time, described the phenomenon of "automaticity" in their article "The Unbearable Automaticity of Being" (*American Psychologist,* July 1999): Goals do not require an act of will to operate and guide information processing and behavior. They can be activated instead by external, environmental information and events.

Once they are put into motion, goals operate just as if they had been consciously intended.

What this means for you is that the more you become conscious of and practice the strategies you'll be learning, the more automatic they will become, to the point where you no longer have to think about thinking. You'll be able to visualize and anticipate events and circumstances and respond to them with the automatic behaviors you already have in place. The more you understand why you do what you do, the better your chances will be of overcoming those barriers. But you have to know what you're jumping over before you make the leap.

By now I'm sure you're at least as excited as you've been just before you started any one of the quick-fix diets that have failed you in the past. I can promise you that this time you won't fail.

Before we begin, I'd like you to go find a small notebook you can use to write down and collect all the information you'll be gathering as we go through the exercises in this book. Once you've done that, we'll get going—and take it one day at a time.

◄◄◄ STEP 2 ►►►

Create a "Livable" Diet

"Great things are not done by impulse, but by a series of small things brought together." —Vincent Van Gogh

If you're like most of my clients, you're ready for some hard-core, practical advice on what you can do *right now* to start dropping pounds. Or, if you've already lost the weight, you want information and strategies that will keep you in the game for the rest of your life. Not every one of the tools I'll be offering will work for every one of you, but you don't need *all* of them. You need to find the ones that *do* work for you because, as I've been saying, this will be your own personalized livable diet, not a prescription to be followed blindly, whether it makes sense to you or not. Some of what I'm about to show you may also seem obvious or sound like nothing more than common sense—and to some it may be both. But I've found that, for almost all my clients, understanding how to create a Livable Diet is not common sense—it may *make* sense, but it's not common sense. There is a world of difference.

So what *is* a Livable Diet? Simply put, it's a diet you can live with for the rest of your life. Still not sure? Let me ask you a quick question: How long can you hold your breath? If you're good, maybe thirty or forty seconds. So, yes, you can do it, but only for a very short period of time. Well, that's how most people diet—they can do it for a bit, but they can't keep holding their breath forever. What they *can* do, however, is create their own, individual, automatic, livable diet—and so can you. In fact, it's the only thing that can work long term. It worked for me, it's worked for thousands of my clients, and it's supported by countless scientific studies.

* * *

In the *Independent*, a London-based newspaper, Dr. Jane Ogden, a professor of health psychology at King's College London, identified three reasons why most diets are not successful: "confusion about what 'cutting down' actually means for everyday eating; the fact that the minute you deny yourself something you become fixated on that object; and the fact that most diets equal eating boring, 'untasty food.'" Therefore, you need to find out what it means to "cut down" and discover "tasty foods" that are low in calories. If you can do those two simple things, you'll be on the road to creating a livable diet, and I'm going to show you how. Then, if you can gear up your physical activity (Step 6) even a small degree in order to speed up your metabolism and increase your calorie spending, you'll have acquired many of the food and fitness tools you need to lose and/or maintain your weight without changing everything else in your life.

Modest lifestyle changes can amount to enormous weight-loss successes.

When I tell people that, they are immediately skeptical. "But what do I actually need to *do*—what's going to help *me* lose weight and keep it off?" "How do I do *that*?" is almost always the first question I'm asked. They're anxious, concerned, and have plenty of other questions, some of which might be, "What's all this about good fats and bad fats, good carbs and bad carbs; what's the difference and how do I know one from the other?" "Can I cheat on the weekends?" "What am I going to have for a treat?" "What am I going to eat when I go out to dinner?" These are valid questions, and before the end of the next two Steps you will have the answers to all of them as well as a good idea of what you're going to be eating tomorrow, next week, and for the rest of your life.

Creating a Livable Eating Program

The most important factor to consider when you begin to think about creating a livable diet is accommodating your own, *individual, food preferences and your personality when it comes to food.* If you don't do that, you'll be feeling deprived, you'll be suffering, and you won't stick to the diet you've chosen because it won't be satisfying. In fact, the *Journal of Nutrition* reports that taste is the single most important reason people choose the foods they do, and that this is also an important factor for regulating "hunger, satiety, and voluntary food intake." That finding is supported by the work of Lisa Sanders, MD, a researcher from Yale University who has determined that finding your own food preference is a key factor in satisfying hunger and the diet's success.

As we've previously discussed, most diet programs are prescriptive; they ask you to follow *their* program, which works great in the short term. But once you get tired of *their* program, you go back to *your* program. And *your* program of choosing what, when, and how much to eat doesn't work. So what you're going to do is come up with food choices that are acceptable to *you*, that you think you can live with. It's going to be a negotiation process, but unlike most bargaining situations, you will not be negotiating with another person, but with yourself.

Here's an illustration of how you'll be negotiating with yourself and still remain within your comfort zone.

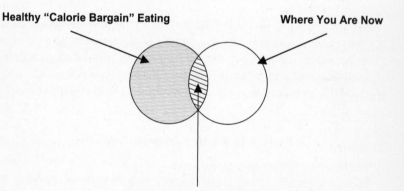

Healthy "Calorie Bargain" Eating   Where You Are Now

Food Choice That Will Work for You Now

The Food Audit: A Three-Day Challenge

Simply by eating one *extra* tablespoon of mayonnaise each day, you will end up gaining about ten pounds in a year—and the reverse is also true. Just by cutting out one tablespoon of mayonnaise, you can lose ten pounds in a year.

Even your smallest food choices matter more than you might ever have thought.

Therefore, the first thing you need to do to create a livable diet is to accept my Three-Day Food Challenge. I challenge you to take a good, hard look at what you eat every day for three full days. The goal: to audit your food choices by keeping track of what you normally eat. Doing this is how you will discover the clues that will allow you to start creating a diet that works. I highly recommend that you write everything down in the notebook I've asked you to get, but if you're not willing to do that (or you don't have your notebook with you), just write on a scrap of paper, or even on the palm of your hand if you have to. Just write it down. I suspect you've probably been asked to keep a food diary before, and the very idea of it may be a real turn-off, *but this is just for three days, and the pay-off will be worth any inconvenience, I assure you.*

I realize, however, that not everyone will be willing to do that. So if you're really opposed to doing my Three-Day Challenge, writing everything down, either because you want to start implementing changes right now, or because you simply don't think you need to, well that's okay (at least for now). In that case, do the Alternative Three-Day Challenge: Try writing down everything you ate in the past three days from memory. (Keep in mind, however, that people typically underreport what they eat by about 50 percent, so overestimate your portions sizes by about that amount; more on this later.) Either way, you can use the sample food diary and instructions in Appendix A to help you get started.

A Picture Is Worth a Thousand Words

The New York Times has reported that a writer named Tucker Shaw has been photographing every single thing that he eats. He labels the photos with the date, time, place, and food. He's doing it to create a historical record, but what a great idea as a way to keep a three-day food diary. If you don't want to write it down, use a small, digital camera (or even a disposable camera) to take photos of every single thing you eat for three days. Make sure to put down the date, time, place, food, and mood.

The problem with trying to keep a mental list is that your mind can play tricks on you, and you might just forget the little snacks you grabbed on the run, the candy you took off your office-mate's desk, or whatever else it might be that you really didn't want to remember. And writing things down will also give you a permanent record to consult when you begin the negotiating process.

Also, keep in mind that while you're taking either Challenge, you don't change your eating habits just yet; all you should be doing is becoming aware and keeping track of them. If you start to change what you eat just because you're noticing it, you won't be creating a realistic starting point.

Small Things Make a Big Difference

When you think about weight gain, you probably think about overeating to excess—whole boxes of cookies, pints of ice cream, or large bags of chips. In reality, however, saving no more than one hundred calories a day can make the difference between weight gain and loss. And that doesn't mean throwing out everything you've got in your kitchen cabinets or turning your life upside down. It means eating one less slice of bread or tablespoon of butter, or cutting out one third of a Snickers bar.

In the journal *Science*, Dr. James Hill, from the University of Colorado Health Science Center, using data from national health surveys, found that cutting one hundred calories per day could prevent weight gain in most of the US population. He and many other health professionals, as well as thousands of my clients, understand that these small changes do make a difference. And the US government has, incidentally, come to this same conclusion. After spending millions of dollars on research, they are launching the Small Steps campaign to help people make the small changes that can have significant impact on their weight. Doing that is certainly one of the components of achieving permanent weight loss, but, in fact, you'll really need *all* the steps in this book to help you maintain your weight loss for life.

What's in a Calorie . . .

If you still have trouble understanding the value of a calorie, keep this in mind: You have to walk an additional twenty-five minutes to burn off each and every one hundred extra calories you eat each day. Now at least you'll have something to relate to the next time you reach for that second bite of cake.

According to CNN, the average American gains about two pounds a year. Since every pound of body weight equals 3,500 calories, two pounds translates into eating only nineteen calories more than you burn every day over the course of a year. So saving one hundred calories would add up to a ten-pound loss per year. You do the math: 3,500 calories equals about a pound; one hundred calories per day is 36,500 calories per year. Divided by 3,500, that's just over ten pounds. Ten pounds may not sound like a lot to you, but it's a good place to start, and it will certainly add up if you can do it year after year without suffering—which is, after all, the whole point.

Here are a few examples of simple substitutions:

▸ Four ounces of water-packed solid white tuna (140 calories) instead of oil-packed (180 calories)
▸ Two cups of skim milk per day (198 calories) instead of two cups of whole milk (304 calories)
▸ Four egg whites (68 calories) instead of two whole eggs (162 calories); or mix 1 whole egg with one egg white (98 calories)
▸ Twelve ounces of diet soda (0 calories) or unsweetened iced tea instead of twelve ounces of soda (160 calories)
▸ One tablespoon of mustard (6 calories) on your sandwich instead of one tablespoon of mayonnaise (100 calories)
▸ Two ounces fat-free bologna (40 calories) instead of two ounces regular (178 calories)
▸ Eight-ounce glass of Tropicana Light 'n Healthy Orange Juice (70 calories) instead of eight ounces of regular orange juice (110 calories)

Health Food Can Also Pack on Pounds

My client Jackie was a health nut. She shopped only in the health-food store and bought organic foods. She ate a vegetarian diet, took loads of vitamins, and preached (to anyone who would listen) about the virtues of eating "pure and healthy." Yet, at thirty-four years old she was fifty-five pounds overweight. Jackie ate *plenty* of health foods. The problem was that she ate them to excess. Many foods give the appearance of being healthy, but actually pack in quite a few calories, fats, and carbohydrates—just stroll down the aisle at Whole Foods or Wild Oats, and really examine some of the food labels. You may be a little surprised by what you discover. For Jackie, the calories added up, and the pounds followed.

When she came to me, she didn't want to hear about any of that "mumbo-jumbo behavior stuff." She was a perfect example of someone who had detached herself emotionally from her eating problems. Looking at her behavior was still too painful! Instead, she insisted that weight control was only about food and blamed her extra pounds on a slow metabolism and twelve-hour shifts at the hospital where she worked.

Jackie constantly cited studies from the latest news headlines: "nuts are healthy"; "a recent study shows that eating a slice of pizza once per day can lower your risk of certain cancers"; "chocolate may ward off heart disease"—and the list goes on. In reality, however, she was simply eating too much of the "right" foods, and some of the "wrong" foods as well. She used olive oil to stir-fry her foods, but the food was swimming in oil. Yes, there have been studies to show that some of the foods she was eating have health benefits, but they still have calories. To Jackie, however, reading that a slice of pizza once a day can lower the risk of certain cancers affirmed her *desire* to have a slice—and not once in a while, but every day.

We solved Jackie's eating problem by making her aware that eating natural or healthy foods doesn't necessarily help you lose weight. People often confuse eating "health foods" with eating *healthily* in order to lose weight and *be* healthy. When I showed Jackie the following information about some of the healthy foods she was eating excessively, she was finally able to understand that she was eating well—but eating too well.

Rice Cakes

Believe it or not, these are still very popular among dieters. Their taste has improved over the years, but to me rice cakes are still the closest thing to flavored cardboard with calories. The food label of Hain's Honey Nut Rice Cakes says that one cake is fifty calories, 0 g fat, and 11 g carbs—but how many of them do we really eat?

Don't get me wrong—if you compare rice cakes to a bag of potato chips, they're definitely better. The problem is that rice cakes are not nutrient dense, which means you don't get a lot, nutritionally speaking, for your consumption, and you will most likely remain hungry.

- ▸ Quaker Nacho Cheese Crispy Minis (nine mini-cakes): 70 calories, 2.5 g fat, 11 g carbs

- ▸ Quaker Chocolate Crunch Rice Cakes (one cake): 60 calories, 1 g fat, 12 g carbs

- ▸ Lundberg Nutra-Farmed Brown Rice Cake (one cake): 70 calories, 0 g fat, 15 g carbs

- ▸ Lundberg Nutra-Farmed Buttery Caramel Rice Cake (one cake): 80 calories, 0.5 g fat, 18 g carbs

Frozen Yogurt

Yogurt has gained a reputation for being a healthy food for a variety of reasons, including improved digestion, prevention of intestinal infection, and reinforcement of immune function. But, regardless of the truth of these claims, we can't ignore the fact that frozen yogurt still contains calories and quite a lot of sugar. And since many of us eat way too many calories as it is, any potential benefits from eating too much yogurt may be negated by the increased health risk of being overweight.

In fact, frozen yogurt, which is typically on a dieter's shopping list, may not have the same health benefits as regular yogurt, and in terms of calories, it is often closer to ice cream than yogurt. Nonfat frozen yogurt might seem like a blessing, but just because it doesn't have fat doesn't mean it's calorie-free. Nonfat frozen yogurt can still contain plenty of calories and carbohydrates. When manufacturers cut fat in a product, they need to come up with some way to keep the flavor, which often means adding additional sugar. Check the labels on low-fat products in your supermarket, and you'll notice the trend.

▶ Häagen-Dazs Strawberry Cheesecake Frozen Yogurt (one cup): 460 calories, 12 g fat, 72 g carbs

▶ Ben & Jerry's Half-Baked Frozen Yogurt (one cup): 420 calories, 7 g fat, 78 g carbs (a bit better than their Half-Baked Ice Cream counterpart, which has 560 calories, 28 g fat, 68 g carbs per cup)

▶ Ben & Jerry's Chocolate Fudge Brownie Low-Fat Frozen Yogurt (1 cup): 380 calories, 5 g fat, 72 g carbs

▶ Edy's Heath Toffee Crunch Frozen Yogurt (one cup): 240 calories, 8 g fat, 36 g carbs

Also, keep an eye on yogurt-covered snacks; some varieties are more like candies in disguise!

▶ One cup yogurt-covered peanuts: 921 calories, 63 g fat, 72 g carbs

▶ One cup yogurt-covered raisins: 750 calories, 22 g fat, 139 g carbs

▶ One cup yogurt-covered pretzels: 391 calories, 14 g fat, 61 g carbs

Veggie Chips

Amazingly, some of these snacks taste great—even better than the so-called fattening ones—but there's a reason why. Most of the time you may save a few calories or fat grams, but in the long run, you may end up eating foods you would never normally eat at all. For instance, I really like Stacy's Simply Naked Baked Pita Chips, which are just slightly lower in calories and fat than potato chips. However, I would never eat potato chips in the first place, and with these, I find myself eating at least half the bag—about 390 calories, 12 g fat, and 54 g carbs. That's the equivalent of eating three bananas or five apples—but at least with the fruit, you get some real health benefits, and also feel more satisfied.

Then there are those Terra Chips. They look so healthy, packaged beautifully, and again, they are lower in calories than potato chips, but are they REALLY good for you? Just one ounce contains 140 calories, 7 g fat, and 18 g carbs—but have you ever heard that advertisement, "Bet you can't eat just one"? It may not be for Terra Chips, but the advertisement still hits the nail on the head.

▸   Good Health Veggie Stix (3 oz): 420 calories, 21 g fat, 54 g carbs

▸ Pirate's Booty (3 oz): 384 calories, 15 g fat, 54 g carbs

▸ Kettle Five Grain Yellow Corn Tortilla Chips (3 oz): 420 calories, 18 g fat, 54 g carbs

▸ Kettle Organic Sweet Brown Rice & Black Bean Tortilla Chips (3 oz): 360 calories, 18 g fat, 48 g carbs

Other Not-So-Healthy Health Foods

Even healthy muffins can make you fat. Although loaded with wholesome ingredients like bran, apples, and oats, they can, in reality, be no "healthier" than a piece of cake! One large muffin with fruit or nuts (3½ inches in diameter): 393 calories, 9.2 g fat. Even low-fat muffins have about 370 calories.

And here are a few others to look out for:

▸ Trail mix (1 cup): 693 calories, 44 g fat, 67 g carbs

▸ Granola (1 cup): 518 calories, 27 g fat, 59 g carbs

▸ Even low-fat granola can contain as many as 427 calories, 6 g fat, 88 g carbs

▸ Balance Bar (1 bar: 50 g): 200 calories, 6 g fat, 22 g carbs

▸ Kashi GOLEAN Chocolate Almond Toffee Bar (1 bar: 78 g): 290 calories, 6 g fat, 45 g carbs

▸ A Snickers bar, just for comparison, contains (1 bar: 58.7 g): 280 calories, 14 g fat, 35 g carbs. That's not a very big difference at all.

▸ Carob chips (1 cup): 934 calories, 54 g fat, 97 g carbs

▸ Banana chips (1 cup): 264 calories, 5 g fat, 60 g carbs. Banana chips are actually no better than potato chips, simply because they are fried.

▶ Dried fruit: Any dried fruit is high in calories because of the high concentration of sugar. One cup of dried apricots, for example, contains 244 calories, 2 g fat.

▶ Nuts are healthy and important in a balanced diet, but that shouldn't give you a license to overindulge. If you add nuts to your diet without decreasing calories from other sources, those extra calories will negate the health benefits by leading to weight gain. The idea is to substitute five or six nuts for some other fat source in your diet, not to add nuts without removing anything else.

▶ And finally, health cookies: Newman's Own Organic Low-Fat Fig Newmans (2 cookies): 130 calories, 2.5 g fat, 26 g carbs; Newman's Own Organic Fig Newmans, Wheat and Dairy Free (2 cookies): 120 calories, 1.5 g fat, 26 g carbs.

Jackie came up with a plan for limiting her portions of healthy food, avoided the phony health food, and also found other foods that were not only healthy, but more filling and lower in calories. So, yes, there are foods that are natural, that may be made from organically grown ingredients, and that are also nutrient dense—like, say, organic vegetable soup. Like Jackie, you need to find your own Calorie Bargains, foods that are both low in calories and satisfying *for you.*

Identify Your Calorie Bargains

For many of us, discount shopping has become a way of life. We look for bargains in clothing, appliances, food, and cleaning products. We go to discount drug stores and wait until things go on sale so that we can get more for less. In fact, I see people in supermarkets all the time carrying a fistful of coupons and comparing the price of one brand to another. There's nothing wrong with that, but I wish more people would put some of their bargain-hunting know-how into shopping for food that will help them create a livable diet. We need to start looking for Calorie Bargains—and by that I *don't* mean buying more food for less money. I mean foods relatively low in calories that taste great and satisfy your strongest temptations.

Generally speaking, when something tastes really good to us we're going to eat more of it. Today, there are plenty of great-tasting foods to be had, but most of them are highly processed (which makes them easier to eat) and pack a lot of calories in relation to their weight or bulk. So what we need to do is find foods that taste good to us, but have fewer calories by weight so that we can eat more of them. Finding them may take some effort, but it can also be fun, and once you've found the Calorie Bargains that work for you, you'll be set for life.

Go to the supermarket when you're not in a hurry, take along a notebook and a pencil, and start the hunt. Compare labels and look for foods you enjoy that are low in calories, fat, and carbohydrates. Pick one that you think you're going to like and take it home for a taste test. You need to be sure it's something you'll enjoy because you're going to be using it to *replace* something else in your diet.

A typical bargain is something that's going to give good value with relation to the price, so when you translate this to food you really need to know how valuable a food will be to you in terms of its satisfaction before you can determine whether or not it's a bargain.

Protein Can Help You Maintain Weight Loss— It's a Good Calorie Bargain

Researchers at Maastricht University in The Netherlands report that a 20 percent higher protein intake, that is 18 percent of total daily calories consumed vs. 15 percent of total daily calories consumed, during weight maintenance, after weight loss, resulted in a 50 percent lower body weight regain, and more lean muscle.

Thomas, a client of mine, loved Ben & Jerry's ice cream so much that he ate it for dessert at practically every meal. After looking at the results of his Three-Day Food Challenge, he realized that this was one place he felt he could compromise. He enjoyed his ice cream, but he figured it was worth a try, so I suggested that he go to the market and buy every single low-calorie ice cream available. He realized this would be a bit expensive, but with all the money he'd already spent on diet supplements, diet books, commercial weight-loss programs, and medical bills, it started to look like an inexpensive solution. In the end, he went home with ten different kinds of low-calorie ice creams and yogurts, and after tasting them all, he decided there were two that would do the trick. When I asked him if they were as good as Ben & Jerry's, he laughed and assured me that no low-calorie ice cream would ever be as good as the full-fat, full-calorie version, but that he could be very happy with his choices for "a very long time" and never feel deprived.

Thomas's ice cream Calorie Bargain allowed him to save about 200 calories a day, and he lost eighteen pounds in a year. Did he compromise? Of course he did. But he didn't feel deprived, he remained within his comfort zone, and because of that he knew he could live with the compromise for life instead of just for the few short weeks he'd have given up ice cream altogether on a quick weight-loss diet.

Keep in mind that this was not a prescription, and Thomas didn't conform to another diet—he came up with something that worked specifically for him. And remember that not all Calorie Bargains come from packaged foods; they can also be found in the foods you cook and those you eat in restaurants. If you tend to eat out frequently and in the same restaurants, it would help to look for the bargains available at those eateries. I will talk more about finding Calorie Bargains in restaurants in Step 3.

Following are a few examples of Calorie Bargains I've been told about by clients and readers of my columns as well as some of my own. For a list of more Calorie Bargains, turn to Appendix B.

Laughing Cow Light, Creamy Swiss Original

One wedge (¾ ounce): 35 calories, 2 g fat, 1 g carbs. Clients (and everyone I tell about this) say the taste is off the charts, and the best part is that one or two wedges will satiate even the insatiable. This cheese is also perfect for the modified low-carb dieter who is looking for low carbs *and* low fat.

Guiltless Potato Fries

One medium baking potato (3" diameter): 133 calories, 0 g fat, 31 g carbs.

Flavored bread crumbs (1 tablespoon): 28 calories, 0 g fat, 5 g carbs.

* * *

Okay, so they're not really fried, but they are just as good as fries, and maybe even better because there's no dieter's remorse. I realize the carbs are a bit high for those on an low-carb program, but these fries are so filling and low in calories that it's worth eating them to prevent other cravings. (But remember, they should be considered a treat and eaten in combination with other foods so that they don't cause a spike in your blood sugar.) Here's how you make them:

Preheat oven to 450 degrees.

Scrub and wash one baking potato. Slice into eighths lengthwise.

Cover a baking sheet with aluminum foil, and spray the foil lightly with cooking spray (e.g., Pam).

Place potato wedges on the tray, and mist the potatoes with cooking spray.

Sprinkle with onion powder, garlic powder, onion flakes, salt, pepper, and paprika. Then sprinkle with one tablespoon of flavored bread crumbs. Reapply a light coat of cooking spray, and bake for approximately 40 to 45 minutes, or to desired crispness. Spray with a light coating of I Can't Believe It's Not Butter spray before serving.

Swiss Miss Diet Hot Cocoa with Calcium

One envelope: 25 calories, 0 g fat, 4 g carbs. It's ideal if you're craving chocolate, and it uses Splenda as the sweetener, so there is no aspartame. How can you go wrong with only 25 calories for hot chocolate?

Homemade Garlic or Herb Toast

One slice low-calorie bread such as Pepperidge Farm Light Style Oatmeal Bread (45 calories, 0 g fat, 9 carbohydrates per slice), five quick sprays of I Can't Believe It's Not Butter spray, and garlic powder or herbs. This snack has gotten clients (and myself) through some rough craving times. Cut it up into strips and you'll feel like you're cheating by eating great-tasting garlic bread. Every time I make this for people, they're amazed at how delicious it tastes—and then they're blown away when I reveal that it's low in calories and fat.

Save a Penny, Gain a Pound, or, Sometimes Cheap Is Dear

Buying ten kinds of ice cream to find one that you like may at first sound to you like a waste of money rather than a bargain, but it's really important that your bargains be foods you like, and there's no way of knowing that until you've tasted them. If Thomas had bought just one kind of low-cal ice cream and didn't like it, he might not have looked any further, and then he'd never have saved those 200 calories a day or lost those pounds. In the long run, spending a little to save a lot really is a bargain, especially when you consider how much money you've already spent on diet products, programs, and books.

And the same goes for foods you don't like. If you don't really like it you shouldn't be eating it, even if you've already paid for it. If you eat it and gain weight, you'll be paying twice, so, when it comes to Calorie Bargains, it doesn't always pay to be thrifty.

Learn to Get Good Value

You have to learn to know a good thing when you see it. Understanding value in food is important, and it's important to think before you eat. Take a look at the following common Calorie Bargains. But *remember,* these are only to be used to *replace* something that you are already eating on a regular basis. A Calorie Bargain should *never* be added to your existing diet; It is only a replacement for higher fat and higher calorie foods. And if it doesn't satiate you, a Calorie Bargain can easily turn into a Calorie Rip-off, which means you'll end up eating more food, consuming more calories, and gaining more weight. So be careful.

Experiment, negotiate, and keep track of you're failures and successes. Your initial goal should be to reduce your calorie intake by 100 to 200 calories a day for maintenance, and about 250 to 400 calories per day for weight loss. This means you should substitute at least 20 percent of your current diet with Calorie Bargains for weight loss and 10 percent of your current diet for weight maintenance. As you become a skilled detective, however, you'll be able to find even bigger bargains.

Instead of: A Big Mac, large fries, and large Coke: 1,450 calories, 59 g fat, 204 g carbs

Save 360 calories with: A Quarter Pounder, medium fries, and medium Coke: 1,090 calories, 43 g fat, 153 g carbs

or even better, save 830 calories with: A Chicken McGrill, small fries, and large Diet Coke: 620 calories, 27 g fat, 65 g carbs

Still better, save 1,025 calories with: A Chicken McGrill, side salad, and large Diet Coke: 425 calories, 17 g fat, 42 g carbs

Best-case scenario, save 1,153 calories with: 2 Chicken McGrills (no bun, no mayo), a side salad with low-fat dressing, and a large Diet Coke: 297 calories, 9 g fat, 15 g carbs

Instead of: A Häagen-Dazs Caramel Pecan Nut Cluster Ice Cream Bar: 420 calories, 16 g fat, 31 g carbs

Save 140 calories with: A Klondike Original Bar: 280 calories, 19 g fat, 24 g carbs

Or even better, save 260 calories with: A Good Humor Chocolate Eclair Bar: 160 calories, 8 g fat, 20 g carbs

Or still better, save 340 calories with: A Häagen-Dazs Chocolate Sorbet Bar: 80 calories, 0 g fat, 20 g carbs

Best-case scenario, save 360 calories with: A Fudgsicle: 60 calories, 1 g fat, 11 g carbs

Instead of: Nachos with the works (cheese, beef, beans, sour cream): 1,704 calories, 105 g fat, 138 g carbs

Save 1,358 calories with: Nachos with cheese and salsa: 380 calories, 19 g fat, 44 g carbs

Or even better, save 1,540 calories with: Chips (1 cup) and salsa (½ cup): 164 calories, 7 g fat, 24 g carbs

Instead of: Movie-theater popcorn with butter (medium): 1,170 calories, 90 g fat, 70 g carbs

Save 690 calories with: Smart Food White Cheddar Cheese Popcorn (3 cups): 480 calories, 30 g fat, 42 g carbs

Or better, save 717 calories with: Caramel-coated popcorn (3 cups): 453 calories, 13 g fat, 83 g carbs

Or even better, save 951 calories with: Oil-popped popcorn with butter (3 cups): 219 calories, 14 g fat, 22 g carbs

Best-case scenario, save 1,078 calories with: Air-popped popcorn (3 cups): 92 calories, 1 g fat, 19 g carbs

Instead of: Hellmann's Real Mayonnaise (3 tablespoons): 300 calories, 33 g fat, 0 g carbs
Save 150 calories with: Hellmann's Light Mayonnaise (3 tablespoons): 150 calories, 15 g fat, 3 g carbs
Or even better, save 225 calories with: Hellmann's Just 2 Good Reduced Fat Mayonnaise (3 tablespoons): 75 calories, 6 g fat, 6 g carbs
Or still better, save 270 calories with: Smart Beat Nonfat Mayonnaise Dressing (3 tablespoons): 30 calories, 0 g fat, 9 g carbs
Best-case scenario, save 285 calories with: Grey Poupon Country Dijon Mustard (3 teaspoons): 15 calories, 0 g fat, <1 g carbs

Instead of: Wendy's Bacon and Cheese Baked Potato: 560 calories, 25 g fat, 67 carbs
Save 140 calories with: Wendy's Plain Baked Potato, with reduced fat margarine (3 tablespoons): 420 calories, 17 g fat, 61 g carbs
Or even better, save 220 calories with: Wendy's Sour Cream and Chives Baked Potato: 340 calories, 6 g fat, 62 carbs
Best-case scenario, save 399 calories with: Guiltless Fries—cut up a baked potato, spray it with Pam and sprinkle with flavored bread crumbs (1 tablespoon), and bake for 45 minutes: 161 calories, 0 g fat, 36 g carbs

---

More Calorie Bargains

Use Spices and Flavors to Make Vegetables and Low-Calorie Foods Taste Great: low-calorie, low-fat, butter-flavoring products, low-calorie sugar substitutes (aspartame, sucralose), lemon or lime juice, flavoring extracts (vanilla, almond, etc.), herbs and spices, horseradish, marinades (make sure to check the label to make sure they're low calorie), soy or Worcestershire sauce (high in sodium), mustard, vinegar, and garlic.

Beverages: water, sugar-free soft drinks, carbonated water, coffee or tea, black or with skim milk and a sugar substitute.

If you need even more ideas for Calorie Bargains, take a look at Dr. Howard Shapiro's *Picture Perfect Weight Loss* and *Picture Perfect Weight Loss 30 Day Plan*. These books, which use dramatic photos to make food comparisons, are a great resource for comparing and substituting foods.

Low-Calorie Cooking: Most of these books have the nutritional information available along with the recipe.

▶ *The Johns Hopkins Cookbook Library Recipes for Weight Loss* by Lawrence J. Cheskin, MD. Lora Brown Wilder Rebus, Inc.: June 2003

▶ *American Heart Association One-Dish Meals: Over 200 All-New, All-in-One Recipes* by American Heart Association. Clarkson Potter: November 2003

▶ *The Golden Door Cooks Light & Easy: Delicious Recipes from America's Premier Spa* by Michel Stroot. Gibbs Smith Publisher: May 2003

▶ *The Golden Door Cookbook* by Michel Stroot (Author). Broadway Books: September 1997

▶ *Conscious Cuisine: A New Style of Cooking from the Kitchens of Chef Cary Neff*. Sourcebooks Trade: October 2002

Soup Can *Sometimes* Help You Lose Weight

Ahhh, a good, hot bowl of soup—not to sound like a commercial, but it brings back fond memories of coming in from shoveling snow to find my mom waiting with a steaming bowl of chicken soup. It warmed me up quickly and was just enough to take the edge off until dinner was ready.

In fact, soup is a great Calorie Bargain if you're looking for something to fill you up. "Because soups have a water base, they tend to make you feel less hungry, and you eat less as a result—which is certainly very helpful in terms of losing weight," says Barbara Rolls, PhD, Professor of Nutrition, Penn State University and author of *The Volumetrics Weight-Control Plan*. Dr. Rolls led a study that found that eating soup prior to your meal could reduce your mealtime consumption by as many as 100 calories. However, "the soup must be fairly low in calories to be the most effective—otherwise you can end up eating two meals," cautions Rolls.

There have been a number of studies showing that soup can help you shed pounds. In one conducted by the Department of Psychiatry and Behavioral Sciences at Johns Hopkins University School of Medicine, tomato soup served as a first course appeared to be more satiating and caused the test subjects to consume significantly fewer calories in their second course than did either melon or cheese and crackers.

But don't run for that ladle just yet—even though they might sound healthy, not all soups are created equal. You have to be aware of what's actually in the bowl. And since most of us don't have time to pull out the saucepan and prepare a homemade pot of soup from scratch, we're left at the mercy of soup from a can or restaurant.

Canned soups, at least, have nutritional information on the label, which is more than can be said for Outback and TGI Friday's, neither of which would even tell us how many ounces of cheese, much less the number of calories or the amount of fat they put in their French onion soup.

Keep in mind that chefs and restaurateurs want to make their food taste great, and most of them are not concerned with *your* waistline. "Although there are many ways for chefs to provide flavorful soups that are low in calories and fat, many resort to the old standby of adding creams, butter, sugar, and excessive amounts of sauces," says Marianne Turow, RD, CHE, professor of nutrition at The Culinary Institute of America.

Here are some tips for choosing super soups, instead of soups that dupe (all serving sizes are 1 cup unless otherwise noted):

The Good

Campbell's Select Chicken Vegetable: 110 calories / 1.5 grams of fat
Campbell's Select Tomato Garden: 100 calories / 0.5 grams of fat
Campbell's Soup at Hand, Hand Blended Vegetable Medley: 88 calories / 1.6 grams of fat (this soup was also a taste favorite in a recent test done by Consumer Reports)

The word *Healthy* is a good rule of thumb. Plenty of the canned soups out there are great for the health conscious, including Healthy Choice, Progresso's 99 percent fat free, and even Campbell's Healthy Request soups. For instance, Healthy Choice New England Clam Chowder has only 110 calories and 1.5 grams of fat. Plus, soups with *healthy* on the label must have less than 480 mg of sodium per serving—a boon when many canned soups have more than 1000 mg per serving.

And the Bad

The further you stray from tomato-based soups or clear soups like vegetable and chicken, the more likely the soup is to be fattening.

Au Bon Pain Lobster Bisque: 250 calories / 18 grams of fat
Denny's Cream of Broccoli Soup, bowl: 574 calories / 43 grams of fat
Denny's New England Clam Chowder, bowl: 624 calories / 42 grams of fat
Creole Gumbo (chicken, sausage, and shrimp): 300 calories / 20 grams of fat
Tom Kha Gai (Thai coconut chicken soup): 355 calories / 36 grams of fat
Hot and Sour Soup: 210 calories / 10 grams of fat

Watch Out for the "Extras"

Just one cup (a handful) of seemingly low-calorie oyster crackers or saltines contains 195 calories and 5 grams of fat, while croutons have about 186 calories and 7 grams of fat. And don't fall for this trap: Au Bon Pain has soup bowls that are actually made of bread—believe it or not, the bowl alone, without any soup, has 600 calories and 2.0 grams of fat!

Creating Your Own Calorie Bargains

Now that you've learned to read labels and steer clear of Calorie Rip-offs, it's time to start looking for bargains of your own. Remember that you need to make sure they're low in calories, fat, and carbs. Okay, now it's time to get out your notebook and do some sleuthing. Here's a sample of the factors to consider when you're choosing a Calorie Bargain for yourself:

Serving Size You Would Eat in a Typical Sitting. Be Honest (measure your worst-case scenario) _____ Okay, now your Total Calories _____ Total Fats _____ Total Carbohydrates _____

Why is this a good choice for you? _____
What other foods would this replace? _____

How are you going to make sure that you will choose this Calorie Bargain over other food choices? _____

Will it do the job of replacing something else in your diet? (1 = highest possible score—it's as good as the food you'll be replacing. 10 = the lowest possible score—you will get bored quickly and feel as if you're on a diet.)

Putting It All Together—Making the Substitution

Instead of _____: _____ calories,
_____ g fat, _____ carbs

Save _____ calories with _____:
_____ calories, _____ g fat, _____ g carbs,

or even better, save _____ calories with _____:
_____ calories, _____ g fat, _____ g carbs

or still even better, save _____ calories with _____:
_____ calories, _____ g fat, _____ g carbs

What's a Cup of Coffee?

Just putting milk and/or sugar in your tea or coffee can add up to quite a few calories.

▶ Half-and-half: (⅛ of a cup or 2 tablespoons) 39 calories
▶ Whole Milk: (⅛ of a cup or 2 tablespoons) 19 calories
▶ Skim Milk: (⅛ of a cup or 2 tablespoons) 11 calories
▶ Sugar: 16 calories per teaspoon

Just three cups of coffee with two tablespoons of half-and-half and two teaspoons of sugar could add up to 213 calories a day or twenty-two pounds in a year.

Try using Equal or Splenda (neither of which is made with saccharin) instead of sugar and skim milk instead of half-and-half.

Many clients constantly upgrade and expand their Calorie Bargains by sharing their discoveries and finding exciting new ways to substitute foods they can live with. Doing this will take some effort, but in the end it can be at least as rewarding as finding a really great bargain on sale in the department store.

Studies on taste preference, according to one published in the *Journal of Public Policy & Marketing*, indicate that people's food preferences are influenced mainly by family—in other words, we tend to prefer foods that we know—but can be broadened if new foods are prepared in a way that is familiar, and that look and taste as we expect them to. In addition, if the main dish in any given meal is rated favorably, the entire meal is usually considered to have been favorable. Because of that, the study suggested that new foods be introduced slowly, as side dishes, and prepared in a way that is familiar.

Try It, You Might Like It

A number of studies have been done on what it takes to get someone to try a new food. Not surprisingly, taste, or the expectation of good taste, ranked high among the reasons people were or were not willing to expand their food choices.

Dr. Paul Rozin, professor of psychology at the University of Pennsylvania, has identified three motivational dimensions for reactions to foods: sensory-affective (liking or disliking taste, smell, or look of food), anticipated consequences (perceived benefits or harm from eating food both immediately or in the long run), ideational (knowledge of food's origins and whether subject will be disgusted or intrigued).

Rozin argues that foods are accepted because they are believed to taste good and have positive benefits, but ideational matters (where the food came from) have little to with food acceptance, but play a factor in rejecting foods. What this means is that people won't eat foods just because they know their source, but can reject foods because of this knowledge; chances are people will reject foods as opposed to trying them once they know where they came from. However, another study showed that once subjects were verbally informed that novel foods tasted good, their willingness to try them increased.

In addition, one study, published in *Appetite*, indicated that when it comes to trying foods based on their nutritional value, "subjects generate no influences to try novel foods because they are good for them, and at times can even be turned off to trying them."

But, says Brian Wansink, PhD, director of the Food and Brand Lab at the University of Illinois, even the pickiest eaters can be taught to try new foods if they're exposed to the food a number of times and not *forced* to eat it. Even children can be taught to expand their food choices, although it may mean getting them to taste the new food ten to fifteen times.

So, the bottom line is, if you hear about or see a new food that looks like a Calorie Bargain, you need to taste it—maybe even fifteen times—to decide if you *really* like it. But don't force yourself to eat it just because it's good for you.

Fill Yourself Up

When you're looking for those compromises and Calorie Bargains that will help to keep you happy without getting fat, the real key is finding foods that will leave you satiated—that is, feeling full and satisfied instead of wanting more. Research has shown that it is indeed possible to consume fewer calories and still feel full. For example, one study conducted by the Nutrition Department at Pennsylvania State University has found that "when individuals were fed diets varying in energy density [that is, number of calories per gram] and could eat as much food as they liked, they ate the same amount of food (by weight), so energy [calories] intake varied directly with energy density. Furthermore, when participants consumed foods of low-energy density, they felt satisfied, despite reductions in energy intake." And Elizabeth A. Bell, another researcher at Pennsylvania State University, also found that women ate a similar weight of food across conditions so that daily calorie intakes varied directly with the calorie density of their diet. They consumed 30 percent less calories daily with the diet of low calorie density than with the diet of high calorie density, although there were no differences in their ratings of hunger and fullness.

The Calorie Bargain Burger

If you use lean instead of regular ground beef (or get even better results by using ground turkey) to make your burger, you'll have the same size burger, but you'll be getting more calories from protein and fewer from fat, and the total number of calories will be lower *even though the burger is the same size.* Or, you could mix regular ground beef with mushrooms, peppers, and onion before forming the burger. Again, you'll have the same size burger, but it will be much lower in calories—and you'll be getting the health benefits of all those vegetables as well.

In addition, the same researchers also found that the effects of volume were dissociated from those of weight. In other words, *you feel full when you get to eat a lot* irrespective of what the food weighs or how many calories it contains (e.g., vegetables). The goal, then, is to look for foods that are large, low in calories, and tasty (so that we are satisfied and want to stop eating).

The amount of fiber and water may have a significant effect on achieving that desired feeling of fullness—which is why soup has been shown to reduce consumption during the balance of the meal.

Make It Low Density

In her groundbreaking book *Volumetrics,* Barbara J. Rolls talks about energy density, or the number of calories with relation to the volume of food, and advises that you eat more foods naturally rich in water, such as fruits, vegetables, low-fat milk, beans, and cooked grains, as well as lean meats, poultry, and fish. She also suggests water-rich dishes like soups, stews, casseroles, pasta with vegetables, and fruit-based desserts.

Water dilutes the caloric density of foods, which means that you get to eat more for less. If, for example, you add water-rich blueberries to your cereal, or eggplant to your lasagne, you'll be adding volume, but few extra calories.

Anne Fletcher, author of *Thin for Life,* has noted that while foods low in fat rate low in satisfaction, foods that are low in fat but high in fiber and water (such as vegetables, fruits, and grains) are more filling because *they take up more room in your stomach and take longer to eat.* Corroborating that finding, a study published in the *American Journal of Clinical Nutrition* reported that consuming food with a high water content effectively reduced subsequent calorie intake.

The bottom line is that eating foods that fill you up will prevent you from overeating later, and those foods are generally the ones that provide the most volume for your calorie buck. The challenge is to reduce the energy density of the foods you choose while still maintaining the taste. The scientific journal *Neuroscience & Biobehavioral Reviews* reported that the most important reason people stop eating is because they become tired of the food, not because they are full. In other words, if you're enjoying the taste, you'll keep on eating even if you're full. So the Calorie Bargains you need to look for are foods you really like that are also low in calories by weight so that you can eat *a lot* without worrying too much about portion control. Portions are certainly important, but if you're having trouble losing weight or maintaining your weight loss, having a few foods in your repertoire that allow you to eat plenty without gaining weight can come in very handy.

To identify a Calorie Bargain—that is, a food you really like, that's low in calories, and that you can substitute for another, more fattening food—you need to become the best diet detective you can be. To do that, so that you can avoid being taken in by a Calorie Rip-off, it's important that you learn to read the nutritional labels that appear on all packaged foods.

Dissecting the Food Label

Food labels are not easy to understand. Believe it or not, the Nutrition Facts panel on the food label is designed to be straightforward. I don't know about you, but I don't find it simple. Nevertheless, you need to be able to decipher the label quickly so that you can start to make substitutions and create your livable diet. If you've been on a diet, you're probably used to reading food labels, but when it comes to saving calories, there are a few important points you really need to keep in mind. Let's start at the top, with the serving size and the number of calories per serving, which is right where the confusion begins.

Nutrition Facts

Serving Size 1 cup (228g)
Servings Per Container 2

Amount Per Serving

Calories 260   Calories from Fat 120

% **Daily Value***

Total Fat 13g	**20**%
Saturated Fat 5g	**25**%
Trans Fat 2g	
Cholesterol 30mg	**10**%
Sodium 660mg	**28**%
Total Carbohydrate 31g	**10**%
Dietary Fiber 0g	**0**%
Sugars 5g	
Protein 5g	

Vitamin A 4%	•	Vitamin C 2%
Calcium 15%	•	Iron 4%

* Percent Daily Values are based on a 2,000 calorie diet.
Your Daily Values may be higher or lower depending on
your calorie needs:

	Calories:	2,000	2,500
Total Fat	Less than	65g	80g
Sat Fat	Less than	20g	25g
Cholesterol	Less than	300mg	300mg
Sodium	Less than	2,400mg	2,400mg
Total Carbohydrate		300g	375g
Dietary Fiber		25g	30g

Calories per gram:
Fat 9   •   Carbohydrate 4   •   Protein 4

Serving Size Matters

Just because the food label lists a certain number of calories per serving does NOT mean that's how much *you* eat. In fact, almost everyone I know consumes much more than the serving size listed on the Nutrition Facts panel. Most people—rather than counting out fifteen chips or measuring a three-ounce serving—either fool themselves into thinking they're eating the right amount or ignore the stated serving size altogether. And because the *entire* Nutrition Facts panel is based on the serving size, it's important to get it right or all the subsequent information will also be inaccurate.

So look at the serving size designated by the manufacturer. Now look at the size of the package. Are you really going to eat only ⅓ cup of that particular item, or will you more likely be eating ½ a cup, or even a cup? If so, you need to multiply the calories by the number of servings you'll actually be eating.

It's been reported in the *New England Journal of Medicine* that people attempting to lose weight tend to *underestimate* the amount they eat by as much as 47 percent and overestimate their physical activity by as much as 51 percent. This is why the Three-Day Food Challenge is so revealing and effective. When scientists at the USDA Human Research Center in Beltsville, Maryland, asked ninety-eight men and women to say how much they ate in a twenty-four-hour period, they found that six out of seven women underreported by 621 calories and six out of ten men underreported by an average of 581 calories. So do be realistic, because if you're not, the only one you'll be fooling is yourself.

A portion of ice cream, for example, is generally listed as one-half cup. Do you know how much that is? If you're not sure, go get a measuring cup out of your kitchen cabinet and take a look. It's probably not as much as you thought.

Have you looked at a box of frozen vegetables lately? They're generally intended to serve three to four. But vegetables are one of the "good" foods on any diet, so don't skimp—just make sure you're being honest with yourself about the amount you're going to eat.

When the American Cancer Institute did a study asking Americans to try to determine the portion sizes of eight specific foods, only 1 percent was able to get it right. Sixty-one percent couldn't get more than four right. To help improve your ability to determine portion size without using a measuring device, take a look at page 242 in Appendix A.

I'm not suggesting you get out a measuring cup or a scale every single time you eat, but it's a good idea to try to get an accurate measurement once in a while. At the very least, measure how much food your bowls, glassware, and plates will hold so that when you fill one, you'll have a good idea of how much you're consuming.

Compare One Label to Another

Comparing one nutrition label to another is one of the best ways there is to find out where you can save on calories.

For example:

One 10-ounce box of frozen broccoli spears = 78 calories

One 10-ounce box of frozen broccoli spears in butter sauce = 144 calories

How about spraying your plain broccoli with I Can't Believe It's Not Butter spray and saving almost half the calories?

One 10-ounce box of corn kernels = 222 calories

One 10-ounce box of spinach = 69 calories

If you like spinach as much as corn, that's a saving of 153 calories, even if you eat the whole box.

Butter vs. Margarine vs. Olive Oil

Did you think all butter was equal? Well think again.

One tablespoon Breakstone's All Natural Salted Butter = 100 calories

One tablespoon Breakstone's All Natural Salted Whipped Butter = 60 calories

One tablespoon Smart Balance 37 percent Light Buttery Spread = 45 calories

Want the taste with even fewer calories?

Twelve sprays I Can't Believe It's Not Butter spray = 10 calories

But be careful.

One tablespoon I Can't Believe It's Not Butter in a tub = 90 calories

One tablespoon margarine = 100 calories

And what about olive oil?

Even though olive oil is heart healthy, it still has 120 calories for one tablespoon. Margarine is a better choice if it has no trans fat for health and calories. (Read on to learn more about trans fat.)

Let Your Fingers Do the Walking

Check out calories, fats, carbs, and more. Search for your Calorie Bargains right in your home—on your computer. Freshdirect.com is a supermarket delivery service in New York City, but you can take advantage of their fabulous Web site no matter where you live. The site offers an impressive amount of nutrition information, arranged in whatever order you choose, for almost every single food in the supermarket. Look for details of every ingredient as well as the Nutrition Facts panel at no charge. Just be sure to input a valid New York City zip code when prompted (try 10011): www.freshdirect.com.

Identifying Calorie Rip-Offs

Reading labels can also show you where compromising would *not* save you calories. This can be particularly useful when you think that switching to a low-fat or low-carb version of a particular food will be helping you to lose weight.

Did you know, for instance, that one serving (two tablespoons) of Skippy Reduced-Fat Peanut Butter has exactly the same number of calories as Skippy Full Fat Creamy Peanut Butter—190. And the reduced-fat version has just four fewer fat grams than the full-fat version. In other words, you'd be better off either way (less fat, fewer calories) by spreading your peanut butter a little thinner and having just one tablespoon instead of two.

Never eat anything with more than 200 calories without taking at least ten seconds to decide if it's really worth it. Is it a Calorie Bargain or a Calorie Rip-off?

A Food Label Alternative: The No Exercise Exercise Diet

Here's one benefit of exercise that doesn't even require you to move a muscle. If you're even thinking of "cheating" or eating something you know you really shouldn't, stop for a minute and consider it in terms of the amount of exercise you'd have to do to burn it off.

For instance, if we were to translate a Twinkie into exercise—it would add up to the equivalent of a thirty-minute walk. The Food and Drug Administration (FDA) could even require food manufacturers and restaurants to put the "exercise equivalent" on the food label. Imagine, a statement right there on the Cinnabon Caramel Pecanbon: "Warning: Eating This Product Could Require an Additional 4 Hours and 10 Minutes of Walking or 5 Hours of Continuous Vacuuming." Just think about the implications. Knowing that we have to walk for fourteen hours at a moderate pace for a distance of roughly forty-three miles in order to burn off one pound of fat—well, that would certainly discourage me from eating. But if we apply it to specific food items—now that could actually work. After all, it's much easier to imagine passing up a double-decker burger with fries, a couple of super-sized Cokes, and a banana split than it is to see yourself out there walking forty-three miles.

The following will help get you started on the No Exercise Exercise Diet:

McDonald's Big Mac, French Fries (large), and a Coke (large)
   Warning: Eating This Product Could Require an Additional 7 Hours of Dog-Walking.

Pizza Hut Stuffed Crust Cheese Pizza (2 slices)
   Warning: Eating This Product Could Require an Additional 1 Hour and 17 Minutes of Jumping Rope.

Hershey's Chocolate Kisses (5 Kisses)
   Warning: Eating This Product Could Require an Additional 15 Minutes of Running.

Hungry Man Fried Chicken Entree (mostly white meat)
   Warning: Eating This Product Could Require an Additional 1 Hour and 9 Minutes of Kickboxing.

The Cheesecake Factory Black-Out Cake (1 slice)
   Warning: Eating This Product Could Require an Additional 3 Hours

and 52 Minutes of Lawn Mowing (and not on one of those riding mowers).

Ben & Jerry's Cherry Garcia Ice Cream (1½ cups)
Warning: Eating This Product Could Require an Additional 2 Hours and 9 Minutes of Riding a Stationary Bike.

Oreo Double Stuf Cookies (3 cookies)
Warning: Eating This Product Could Require an Additional 18 Minutes of Swimming Laps.

Piña Colada (8 oz.)
Warning: Drinking This Product Could Require an Additional 1 Hour and 5 Minutes of Golf, Walking and Carrying Your Own Clubs.

PowerBar Protein Plus (1 bar)
Warning: Eating This Product Could Require an Additional 55 Minutes of Vigorous Dancing.

Fats and Why They Matter

We've come a long way since the days when all fats were taboo. We need fat in our diet—it's recommended that about 25 to 30 percent of our daily food intake come from fat, with limited bad fats and an emphasis on good fats. Barbara J. Rolls, PhD, writing in the *Journal of Nutrition,* reported that "a number of studies have compared the effects of fat and carbohydrate on both satiation (the amount eaten in a meal) and satiety (the effect on subsequent intake), but have found little difference between these macronutrients when the palatability and energy density were similar." Translation: fat does not necessarily cause you to eat more or less, nor does it necessarily affect how quickly you become hungry after eating. Rather, if the energy density (how many calories per gram the food happens to be) and palatability of a fat and a carbohydrate are equal, they will have the same effect on your satiation and satiety. You need some fat to help you feel satisfied, just not as much as you typically eat.

The problem is that fat is expensive. What do I mean by that? Well, every gram of fat costs you about nine calories, whereas every gram of protein or carbohydrate costs four calories. This means that on a gram-for-gram basis, fat calories will add up much quicker than carbs or protein. And when fat is combined with other foods to enhance their tastes, it becomes very easy to consume too many fat calories too quickly (just look at a small piece of chocolate versus an apple). That's why nutritionists and health professionals constantly warn against fat intake. But having no fat is not good either because we need it in our diet for health reasons, as well as for taste. And when you do reduce fat intake, it's not a good idea to replace it with carbohydrates, because they, too, can add up quickly. In terms of health, there are good and bad fats, and you should know the difference.

Good Fats, Bad Fats

The Bad Fats

Saturated Fat: These fats, which are listed on the label, are found primarily in animal products such as meat, whole-milk dairy products, poultry skin, and egg yolks. Consuming too many of these fats can raise your "bad" cholesterol levels; therefore, less than 10 percent of your total calories should be derived from saturated fat.

Trans Fat: This kind of fat was developed to increase the shelf-life of food. To do that, manufacturers blast healthy, polyunsaturated oils with hydrogen gas to solidify them, and, in the process, make them incredibly unhealthy. The problem is that trans fat won't be listed on the label until 2006, so you need to look for trans-fat clues. Learn "suspect" foods, such as margarines (unless they say "no trans fat" on the label), shortenings, deep-fried foods, fast foods, and many commercial baked goods such as pies, cookies, cakes, crackers, and doughnuts. Check the ingredients list, and be on the lookout for partially hydrogenated oil—if it's there, you have trans fat. Also, many products now promote the fact that they are "trans-fat free"—so look for that designation on the front of the packaging.

The Good Fats

"Good" or unsaturated fats are found in products derived from plant sources, such as vegetable oils, nuts, and seeds. There are two main categories.

Monounsaturated: These fats are found in high concentrations in canola, peanut, and olive oils, as well as olives, peanuts and peanut butter, and avocados. There is evidence that monounsaturated fats help lower LDL (the "bad") cholesterol and raise HDL (the "good") cholesterol levels in your body.

Polyunsaturated: These fats are prevalent in sunflower, corn, safflower, cottonseed, and soybean oils, as well as nuts and fish (omega-3). They've been found to help lower total cholesterol levels and prevent heart disease (particularly the omega-3s).

Keep in mind, however, that whether a fat is good or bad it still contains calories. A tablespoon of olive oil still has 120 calories.

Trimming the Fat from Your Recipes

To trim the fat from your favorite recipes, you need to know the role that fat plays in cooking. Fats give foods flavor, texture (also called mouth-feel), richness, and sheen. That's why you can't take out all the fat of most dishes and expect them to taste the same. In order to get the most flavor out of lower-fat recipes, follow these guidelines:

- **Use low-fat cooking techniques:** Bake, broil, steam, or grill rather than fry.
- **Add herbs and spices:** They add a lot of taste with practically no calories. To release their full aroma, always crush them before adding to recipes.
- **Marinate:** Whether it's vegetables, meat, poultry, or fish, marinating adds enormous amounts of flavor. Make sure to marinate tofu, otherwise it will have no taste.
- **Use nonstick cookware:** You can cook just about anything without using any oil at all.
- **Use nonstick cooking spray:** Choose those without hydrogenated oils.
- **Substitute low-fat ingredients for high-fat ingredients:** Use light sour cream, low-fat mayo, light cream cheese, and low-fat cottage cheese.
- **Choose lean cuts of meat:** Round, sirloin, and loin cuts.
- **Remove skin from poultry before you eat:** Cooking with the skin on will retain moisture and keep poultry tender; however, remove it before you eat, and the fat content will be cut in half.

> ▶ Use two egg whites or ¼ cup of a liquid egg substitute in place of one whole egg.
>
> ▶ Replace some of the fat in baked goods with applesauce, mashed bananas, or pureed prunes, pears, peaches, or apricots: Fruit purees mimic many of the functions fat performs in baking. They reduce the need for fat because their fibers and naturally occurring sugars hold moisture in baked goods. They do not, however, provide enough tenderness and must, therefore be used in combination with some fat. Use half the amount of fat called for in the recipe and an equal amount of fruit puree.

Carbohydrates Are Not All Bad

Carbohydrates. Yes, I said the "C" word. I'm amazed at the anger and frustration Americans have toward carbohydrates these days. Perhaps they feel duped by nutrition experts for telling them to replace fat with an abundance of carbs, a recommendation that may be one of the causes for the recent increase in our waistlines.

In fact, the Centers for Disease Control and Prevention (CDC) has found that between 1971 and 2000, the average calorie intake increased 22 percent for women and 8 percent for men, mainly from eating more carbohydrates such as rice, bread, and pasta, as well as pizza, salty snacks, and takeout foods, and from increased portion size.

Carbs are taking a big hit these days, even though they are an important nutrient and necessary for survival. Foods that contain carbohydrates include fruits, vegetables, whole grains, beans and legumes, nuts, milk, and yogurt (the "good" carbs), as well as cookies, cakes, soft drinks, syrups, and, of course, table sugar (the "bad" carbs).

Carbohydrates are broken down into two categories on the food label—dietary fiber and sugar. Dietary fiber does not convert to glucose and thus does not raise your blood sugar the way other carbohydrates typically do, and it makes you feel full longer—a good thing.

The "sugars" section includes those that are present naturally in the food (such as lactose in milk and fructose in fruit), as well as those that are added to the food during processing, such as high-fructose corn syrup. In most cases, your body can't distinguish between the two.

If carbs are so bad, then why were we told to eat more of them in the first place? Recent diet books have been emphasizing the "good" carbs with astonishing success. But how do we know which are the right carbs to eat? And is this really the healthier path in the first place?

Good Versus Bad

The concept of "good" versus "bad" carbs actually derives from the now outdated concept of differentiating complex carbohydrates (i.e., starches) from simple carbohydrates (i.e., sugars). The idea was that simple sugars digest quickly while the longer-chain, complex carbohydrates take longer to digest and, therefore, keep you full.

However, a complex carbohydrate can also be refined (e.g., white bread, white rice, and pasta), a process that strips away much of the good stuff like fiber, vitamins, and minerals. At the same time, there are many simple carbohydrates that are unrefined (e.g., fruits and vegetables) and, therefore, still contain fiber, vitamins, and minerals. So dividing carbs this way is too simplistic to guide your food choices.

That's where the glycemic index (GI) comes in.

Decoding the Glycemic Index

Created as a research tool to determine the actual effect carbohydrates have on blood sugar, the glycemic index measures how quickly a food that contains carbohydrate raises a fasting person's blood sugar and subsequent insulin levels over a two-hour period. (Insulin is the hormone that activates cells to absorb sugar from the bloodstream, thus reducing blood-sugar levels.)

Foods with a high GI value raise the body's blood-sugar levels very quickly, which signals a corresponding rapid release of insulin into the bloodstream that then lowers blood-sugar levels.

In contrast, low-GI meals cause a slower release of sugars into the bloodstream, thus triggering a more moderate insulin release, which allows for the slower metabolism of carbohydrates and supposedly keeps you feeling full longer.

But it isn't that black and white. "There aren't any conclusive studies. The majority of, but not all, one-day studies show low-GI foods suppress hunger, but no relevant long-term studies have been completed," says Christine Pelkman, PhD, professor of nutrition at the

University of Buffalo in New York. "Not only that, there's no proof that following a low-GI diet will aid in weight loss."

Another problem is that there are a multitude of variables—including fiber or fat content, acidity, food combinations, preparation method, and even ripeness—that affect the way your body handles carbohydrates.

And portion size is also an issue. The Index is based on a fifty-gram carbohydrate portion of food, which is significantly more than a typical serving of many foods. Carrots, for example, have a GI of ninety-two, which is much higher than that of many other vegetables. But in order to get fifty grams of carbohydrate you would have to eat about one and a half pounds of carrots—much more than most people would ever consume.

To take the serving size into account, the glycemic load (GL) was introduced in 1997. The GL of a food is equal to that food's GI value multiplied by the number of carbohydrate grams in the portion of food, divided by one hundred. When portion size is taken into account, those carrots take on a GL of between three and four. (For GI/GL values: http://www.glycemicindex.com/.)

In addition, the GI/GL of a food can have nothing to do with whether or not it is high in calories. Take ice cream, for example—a half cup has a GI of 42 and a GL of 7, making it seem almost healthy; but, of course, it's loaded with calories and fat! "If you look at GI/GL all on its own, it might not lead to a healthier or more satisfying diet," says Pelkman. "Soda has a lower GI than carrots, so if you were just using GI, you would choose soda over carrots—these are not choices that would lead to weight loss," she cautions. In a report in *Nutrition Action* published by the Center for Science in the Public Interest, one of the glycemic index's authors, Thomas Wolever, was himself quoted as saying that he believes the index is "no magic bullet for dieters . . . I've yet to see evidence that a low-GI diet aids in weight loss . . . one or two studies show it and a number of others don't." Dr. Wolever then goes on to say that his book *The New Glucose Revolution* is not a diet book despite the "Lose Weight" claim on its cover.

So What Should You Eat?

Most nutrition experts advise eating a diet rich in high fiber foods such as whole grains, vegetables, legumes, and fruit. It's been shown that high-fiber foods do tend to promote weight loss because they are generally bulky and contain a lot of water, two factors that make them low in caloric density. Water, as we've already noted, can fill you without making you fat, and fiber has only 1.5 to 2.5 calories per gram (as opposed to four in carbs and protein or nine in fats). So remember, it's the fiber *in the food* that helps to fill you and thus promote weight loss; taking fiber pills isn't going to make you thin.

Reporting on a study completed at the University of Arkansas, Jane Brody wrote in the *New York Times* that "fiber-rich carbohydrates offer three major benefits to the weight-conscious eater: they hold water in the gut, take longer to digest, and some of their calories are eliminated unabsorbed. In other words, they can fill you up before they fill you out."

"You need to look for low-calorie, low-density foods [the least amount of calories per gram weight] that will satisfy you," says Pelkman. *This is often the food that is the least processed.* Again, pick foods that fall into the following areas: fruits, vegetables, whole grains, lean meats, low-fat milk products (milk, yogurt, hard and soft cheeses), low-fat or fat-free foods or snacks, sugar-free beverages.

Calorie for calorie, foods high in fat will be less satisfying than foods low in fat and high in fiber and water (vegetables, fruits, and grains) because low fat, high-fiber foods take up more room in your stomach and take longer to eat. Keep this in mind: Check the amount of dietary fiber listed on the Nutrition Facts panel of the label, if it's high in fiber, it's a clue that it's a low calorie, low-density food.

Translating the Front of the Label

Even though the Food and Drug Administration (FDA) regulates the use of these terms (known as "nutrient content claims"), the front of the food label can be as complicated to read as the back. Here are a few hints that will help you to avoid Calorie Rip-offs and hunt for the Calorie Bargains.

Low-Fat Lies

Fat-Free: A fat-free food must have fewer than 0.5 grams of fat per serving. The key words here are "per serving." You still have to remember that the manufacturer's serving size may be quite different from the portion you actually eat. I Can't Believe It's Not Butter spray is a good example of how this can be misleading. Even though the label boasts "zero" calories and "zero" fat, that's just for a few sprays. If you use twenty-five sprays, it's actually twenty calories and about two grams of fat—and while that's still low, it's not "zero."

Or, take a look at another popular product—Pam Cooking Spray (one of my longtime favorites). Although Pam has fewer than 0.5 grams of fat per serving, technically qualifying it for the "fat-free" claim, the FDA thought such an assertion on a product that is essentially 100 percent fat (that's right—it's full of fat) would be misleading, so they compromised by allowing Pam (and other, similar products) to put the words "for fat-free cooking" on the label.

And many fat-free foods have almost as many calories as similar foods that are not fat free—usually because the fat has been replaced with additional carbohydrates. Nine Nabisco Snackwell's Fat-Free Wheat Crackers, for example, have 108 calories, 0 grams of fat, and 21.6 grams of carbohydrates, while nine Nabisco Premium Saltine Crackers have 108 calories, 2.7 grams of fat, and 18 grams of carbohydrates.

Low-Fat: To qualify as low-fat, a food must contain three grams of fat or less per serving. (Notice those words again—"per serving.") But that doesn't mean it's necessarily healthy or low in calories.

Ben & Jerry's Chocolate Fudge Brownie Low-Fat Frozen Yogurt, for instance, contains 190 calories, 2.5 grams of fat, and 36 grams of carbohydrates per serving. On the other hand, plain old Breyers Chocolate Ice Cream has 160 calories, 9 grams of fat, and 18 grams of carbohydrates per serving.

Reduced or Less Fat: To qualify as a reduced-fat food, the product must have at least 25 percent less fat per serving than the original version.

At 140 calories and 6 grams of fat per ounce, Sun Chips French Onion flavor is correctly labeled as containing 30 percent less fat than regular potato chips. It does, nevertheless, contain about 38.5 percent fat and does NOT meet the criteria for a low-fat food. If you regularly snack on chips, Sun Chips might make a better choice—but they're certainly not as virtuous as the label suggests. So, if you see a "reduced-fat" claim, be wary—yes, it's reduced, but the question is, from what? And never assume that because the label says reduced fat you can eat larger portions without adding extra calories.

Bitter Sweet

Sugar-Free: When you see this on the front of the label, it means that the product has fewer than 0.5 grams of sugar per serving. But again, that doesn't mean it's necessarily healthy or great for weight loss.

Take a look at Murray Sugar-Free Chocolate Chip and Pecan Cookies, which have 160 calories, 10 grams of fat, and 19 grams of carbohydrates per serving. Compare this to a serving of regular Famous Amos Chocolate Chip and Pecan Cookies at 150 calories, 8 grams of fat, and 19 grams of carbohydrates.

No Sugar Added: "No added sugars" and "without added sugars" claims are allowed if no sugar or sugar-containing ingredient (for example, fruit juices, applesauce, or dried fruit) is added during processing or packing. Pay attention though, because it doesn't mean the food is "low calorie" or even "reduced calorie."

Fruit juice with no added sugar is a good example. The juice itself is still high in calories and naturally high in fruit sugars. Ocean Spray No Added Sugar Cranberry Juice has 100 calories and 25 grams of carbohydrate per serving—only slightly less than Ocean Spray Cranberry Cocktail, which has 109 calories and 27 grams of carbohydrate per serving.

Living Light

Light: "Light" or "lite" products are getting a lot of shelf space these days, but "light" is not synonymous with healthy. A "light" food is one that has ⅓ fewer calories *or* half the fat of a previous version of the food.

A great example is the Milky Way Lite. Talk about technicalities:

Milky Way: 270 calories and 10 grams of fat
Milky Way Lite: 170 calories and 5 grams of fat

Here's the catch—a regular Milky Way weighs 58 grams, while a Milky Way Lite weighs only 44.5 grams. So, basically, you could chop off 13.5 grams of your usual Milky Way with similar nutritional results.

The term "light" can also be confusing because it is used to refer to the color or texture of the product as well as its fat or calorie content. Light olive oil, for example, contains the same amount of fat as any other olive oil—nearly 14 grams per tablespoon.

It's Routine

Even though what we've been discussing is all about saving calories, I'm not suggesting that you're going to have to walk around with a calorie counter in your pocket for the rest of your life. Just the opposite. A study in the *International Journal of Obesity and Related Metabolic Disorders* reports that only 30 percent of those who maintain their weight actually count calories, and Anne Fletcher also indicates in her book *Thin for Life* that those who have truly mastered weight maintenance don't count calories or fat grams, they simply know the kinds of foods (low in fat, lots of fruits and vegetables) they need to eat to fill themselves up and still maintain their weight. And that's exactly what you'll be doing as you, too, become a master of weight maintenance.

As Dr. Judith Ouellette and Dr. Wendy Wood reported in the *Psychological Bulletin:*

> To maintain intentions to adopt a healthier lifestyle, change strategies should ensure that some immediate, positive consequences emerge from the new healthy behavior. In addition, effective strategies should provide the opportunity for repetition of the new behavior in a stable, supporting environment. Frequent performance of the desired behavior in such contexts is especially likely to yield new habits that can themselves proceed relatively automatically.

What that means is, once you've *chosen* to lose weight, and begin to find the Calorie Bargains that work for you, you will experience positive outcomes, which will reinforce your new behavior to the point at which it will become *automatic*. In the following Step we'll be discussing how you can provide yourself with the kind of supportive environment that will help you do that.

◄◄◄ STEP 3 ►►►

Make It Automatic

"Creating a positive environment may lead to success even if a person is not fully motivated, because positive environments help the person retain good habits." —Farrokh Alemi, PhD, *Journal of Healthcare Quality*

"Habit is a compromise effected between the individual and his environment." —Samuel Beckett

You can't control the portion sizes at your local restaurant, or the fact that it's difficult to understand the food label, or that manufacturers put excessive amounts of sugar, fat, or both in the foods you love. But you can control your "personal food environment." The idea is to take responsibility for what you *can* control, and not to leave things to chance. If you were an alcoholic, for example, you probably shouldn't work in a bar, right? Well the same thing goes for eating and being overweight. You need to set yourself up so that you succeed right from the start by altering the way you live—just a bit. Do the work once and it becomes automatic so that over time it will be second nature.

Michael R. Lowe, PhD, a professor in the Department of Psychology at Drexel University, found that creating and monitoring your "personal food environment" is the most effective thing you can do to keep the weight off. "You need to limit your exposure to high-calorie foods in your immediate environment by, for instance, choosing healthier restaurants and stocking your home with quality ingredients and foods," Lowe suggests. Other recommendations include using sugar and fat substitutes and eating more lean protein and fiber-rich foods to increase satiety (gratification beyond the point of satisfaction).

The reason this is so important, he says, is that:

The omnipresence of energy-dense foods in the general environment makes it essential that obesity-prone individuals purposefully engineer the eating-related situations they regularly encounter to ensure that their food selections will be based more on their weight-control needs than on the lure of foods that happen to be available in a given environment. The reason for the emphasis on directly controlling what foods people expose themselves to is that foods are biologically powerful stimuli, and through learning, can become psychologically powerful as well. As such, the appeal of food can easily overpower what people "know" is good for them.

And he's not the only one to think that. In fact, all of my successful clients report that they create "safe" environments and set up a series of comfortable "rules to eat by" around the house, when they go out to eat, at parties, and in their office. And yet, many people still seem reluctant to do that. When asked why, Lowe postulated that we don't like to feel as if we can't control what we eat, and rearranging our environment is tantamount to admitting that food controls us more than we control it.

To make sure that you *are* in control, you need to set yourself up for success. Here's how you can do that.

In Your Home

There are many techniques you can use to help control your weight and develop better "food behaviors," and the best place to start is the kitchen—the "heart" of your food choices.

How Does Your Kitchen Stock Up?

Okay, so what's in your kitchen? You need to know! If you're familiar with what's in your kitchen, it'll be easier for you to come up with ideas for quick meals and healthy snacks.

Get out your notebook, take the following questions with you to your kitchen, and start snooping:

1. How many different kinds of fruit are in your kitchen right now? How about vegetables?
2. How many different varieties of cookies, cakes, or candy? What are they? Are they packaged or homemade?
3. What beverages, other than water, are there to drink?

4. Check out the cereals . . . what kinds are there? Do any of them say "high fiber" or "good source of fiber"? Where is sugar on the ingredient list? (The closer to the beginning of the ingredients list, the more prevalent it is in the food.)

5. What kind of bread is around? What kind of sandwich could you make with the available ingredients if you were looking for a healthy meal?

6. How about good sources of calcium such as dairy products? Can you find any low-fat yogurt or milk?

7. What healthy snacks are in the cabinets or fridge?

8. Do you have an ongoing grocery list posted in your kitchen to write down items that need to be replaced?

Don't Overstock the Pantry

Do you spend more money when you've got more in your pocket? Well, the same seems to be true of your cupboard. According to Brian Wansink, PhD, Director of the Food and Brand Lab at the University of Illinois, "When people with stockpiled levels of soup were asked to recall the last time they ate soup, then asked how much soup they intended to use in the next two weeks, their answers were double that of the normal group." So, don't buy "extras" of foods that tempt you to overeat. And don't buy "fattening" foods just so you'll have them on hand "in case you have company" or for the kids.

Keep in mind that you should also avoid buying packaged foods in large sizes. Why? Larger package sizes encourage greater pouring, which means more eating. According to an article in the *New York Times,* shopping at price clubs, where wholesale-size packages of high-calorie foods are available at very low prices, has contributed to our national obesity epidemic. So here's yet another instance when you might want to rethink the cost/benefit ratio of the amount you spend in the supermarket. Those smaller sizes might cost a few pennies more, but they'll save you pounds, and if you use them more slowly, maybe they're not so expensive after all!

When you're rethinking and restocking your pantry, do it thoughtfully and gradually, a few items at a time. And don't go wild throwing out items you'll just be rebuying when they go on sale in a month. Remember, creating a livable diet is not about overhauling and changing your entire life.

Stocking Up Your Healthy Kitchen

Rethink your shopping list and make sure at least some of the healthful items listed here make it into your cart. Review the list and start by buying a couple of new foods you think you might like to try. Slowly add to your inventory. Remember, variety is the spice of life—with a variety of foods on hand, healthy meals and snacks will be easy to prepare. Nutritious cooking starts with a well-stocked, healthy pantry.

Protein Sources

Pump up your protein intake and watch the fat melt away!

▸ Cheese, fat-free (ricotta)
▸ Chicken breast, skinless
▸ Cottage cheese, fat-free
▸ Deli meat, low-sodium turkey or chicken breast
▸ Eggs and egg whites (use 1 yolk for every three whites)
▸ Fish: flounder, cod, halibut (white fishes)
▸ Nuts and seeds: low-sodium walnuts, almonds, and sunflower
▸ Nut butters—almond and peanut butter (choose 100 percent natural brands)
▸ Pork tenderloin
▸ Protein powder (soy or whey) to make high-protein smoothies
▸ Sausage, low-fat, low-sodium turkey/chicken (in moderation)
▸ Sea steak, such as tuna
▸ Seitan
▸ Shellfish
▸ Soy milk (low-fat)
▸ Steak, extra lean (in moderation)
▸ Ground beef, extra lean (top sirloin, filet)
▸ Tempeh
▸ Tofu, low-fat
▸ Tuna, albacore, low-sodium, packed in water
▸ Turkey breast, whole or ground

Nonstarchy Vegetables

Low in calories, high in fiber, and packed with nutrients, nonstarchy vegetables are your new best friend! Keep some in your freezer so you'll have them on hand to add to soups, stir fries, and pasta dishes. Contrary to popular belief, frozen vegetables are just as nutritious as they were when fresh. Start going to your local farmers' market. You can see what is in season and get some exercise by walking. You may even feel brave and try something new! Many markets now offer pre-washed veggies in bags that are ready to go.

- Artichokes
- Asparagus
- Beans: green, wax, snap peas
- Beets
- Broccoli
- Brussels sprouts
- Cabbage, all types
- Carrots
- Cauliflower
- Celery
- Cucumber
- Eggplant
- Fennel
- Greens: collard, mustard, turnip
- Lettuce: all types
- Mushrooms
- Onions, leeks
- Pea pods
- Peppers: yellow, red, green
- Radishes
- Salsa (fresh)
- Spinach
- Tomato
- Zucchini/summer squash

Healthy Starches

- Whole-grain, high-fiber breads (Ezekiel makes a fantastic one)
- Brown rice
- Whole-wheat, artichoke, or brown-rice pasta
- Beans
- Barley
- Quinoa
- Oatmeal
- Instant rice and couscous: I am sure you're familiar with rice, but couscous may be new to you. It's a quick-cooking ground semolina pasta that's sold plain or already seasoned—all it needs is five minutes on the stovetop. It comes in white and whole-grain varieties and is just as versatile as rice. Try it as a side with chicken, fish, or mixed with veggies.

Other Healthful Helpers!

- Herbs and spices—a calorie-free way to add flavor to your meals! Use fresh or dried. Experiment! You can grow them fresh right in your windowsill. Check out www.herbkits.com and www.mybackyard.com.

▸ Fat-free cooking sprays—an easy way to eliminate fat from your favorite dishes. They now come in a wide variety of flavors.

▸ Flavored olive oils—you only need a small amount for amazing flavor. I make my own using fresh herbs and spices. Make sure to keep in the fridge so that it doesn't turn rancid. It may thicken a bit, but will liquefy quickly at room temperature.

▸ Fat free, low-sodium chicken broth. A great way to cook, bake, roast, simmer, or sauté.

▸ Limes, lemons, and oranges add terrific flavor to any meal without added fat.

▸ Low-sodium soy sauce and ponzu sauce are great additions.

▸ Rice, apple cider, and balsamic vinegars add a lot of zing.

▸ Wasabi paste

▸ Miso paste

▸ Garlic and onions are another way to spice up whatever you're cooking.

▸ Tomato sauce (½ cup, low-fat, low-sodium)

▸ Tomato/vegetable juice (low-sodium)

▸ Stewed tomatoes. It wasn't long ago that I discovered the many uses for this terrific product. Sold in the can, they are inexpensive and add a wonderful taste to many of my favorite meals. I use them most often as an addition to my spicy black beans and rice recipe, but they are also a frequent addition to chicken, chili, and pasta.

▸ Herbal teas and seltzers. These calorie-free beverages are great to have on hand for a tasty way to curb cravings. Add a little lime or lemon.

▸ Unbleached and whole wheat flour

▸ Dried fruit (in moderation)

▸ Sweeteners—aspartame (Equal) or sucralose (Splenda) for a change

▸ Spectrum mayo (a nondairy mayonnaise substitute)

▸ Mustard

▸ Sugar-free ketchup

▸ Low-sodium, low-sugar BBQ sauce

▸ Low-calorie salad dressings (watch for sugar and sodium content)

▶ Applesauce, fruit-juice sweetened

▶ Canned beans, low-sodium

And Here Are a Few Items You Ought to Think About Throwing Out

▶ Soda	▶ White flour
▶ Deli meats	▶ White rice
▶ Full-fat cheese	▶ Pizza
▶ Cookies	▶ Ice cream
▶ Cakes	▶ Butter or margarines with trans fats
▶ Crackers	▶ Chips
▶ Sugary cereals	▶ Maple syrup
▶ Mayonnaise	▶ Lard
▶ White breads	▶ Cake, cookie, brownie mixes

Think of it this way: If you always had a pint of ice cream in the house, you might believe you'd be able to eat it in moderation, but if you're a prime-time TV food eater and your favorite show is about to come on, you will more than likely reach for that pint—why else would it be there?

The trick is to make sure your home (and your office) is fully stocked with Calorie Bargains. Having a supply of snacks and foods that are low in calories is a lot safer than thinking you can simply "wing it" and resist what's there to be had.

Variety Isn't Always the Spice of Life

USA Today reports that Americans are becoming more and more picky—in fact, Dreyer's/Edy's Grand Ice Cream, "which offered thirty-four flavors in 1977, sells 250 today—including options for nut-free, gluten-free, dairy-free and kosher ice cream," "Starbucks . . . has more than 19,000 ways it can serve a cup of coffee," and "Tropicana, which had two kinds of orange juice just a decade ago, now has twenty-four."

Variety may be the spice of life, but when it comes to making food choices, the more we have available to us the worse off we are. If you hadn't already figured that out for yourself, a study conducted by Megan A. McCrory, PhD, and published in the *American Journal of*

Clinical Nutrition concluded that, "a high variety of sweets, snacks, condiments, entrées, and carbohydrates, coupled with a low variety of vegetables promotes long-term increases in energy intake and body fatness." The more "bad choices" you have available to you, the more likely you are to succumb to their temptation. In fact, one of the reasons why diets work at all is because they narrow the variety of allowable foods, limit your choices, and make food intake much more manageable.

But variety in general can also increase the amount you eat. Both Barbara Rolls and Brian Wansink have investigated the effect of variety on consumption, with very similar results. When Rolls offered people sandwiches with four different fillings, they ate one-third more than when she offered them sandwiches with only their single, favorite filling. Similarly, Wansink found that when given jelly beans in six colors, people ate about 40 percent more than when they were given just four colors.

The exceptions: People who eat a variety of fruits and dairy products have no more (or less) body fat than those who eat only one or two varieties. And people who eat the widest variety of vegetables have less body fat than others. Vegetables are good news for people who are trying to reduce their weight. They're low in calories and density, so they may displace calorie-dense foods, and their bulk will reduce overeating.

Cut Out Liquid Calorie Rip-offs

Even 100 percent juice has real calories—in most cases, it has the same number of calories as soda (about 160 calories for twelve ounces), sweetened iced tea, and fancy coffee drinks. Think about it: five or six oranges had to be squeezed to make one glass of juice—so you're getting the sugar from all those oranges.

A study by Richard Mattes, MPH, PhD, RD, a researcher at Purdue University, has reported that people did not compensate for extra liquid calories at all. Fifteen normal-weight men and women were given an extra 450 calories a day as either a liquid (three 12-ounce cans of soda) or a solid (45 large jelly beans) for four weeks each, and those who had the liquids tended to eat more and increased their body weights. *Make sure to keep calorie-free beverages like sparkling or flat water, diet soda, and unsweetened iced tea in your home, office, and car. Replace one twelve-ounce soda with a diet soda each day and drop more than fifteen pounds in one year!*

The Key to Healthier Cooking

Sometimes how you cook your food is as important as *what* you cook. As you now know, virtually all fruits and vegetables are natural Calorie Bargains, low in fat and high in fiber and water. And protein also gives good value (four calories per gram, whereas fat is nine calories per gram). The trick is to cook these (and all) foods so that you don't *add* all the fat they naturally lack. Here are a few kitchen gadgets and appliances to help cooking healthfully become automatic.

Kitchen Fitness

Cooking Spray or Oil Mister:

Since all oils contain about 120 calories and fourteen grams of fat per tablespoon, using an oil mister or cooking spray can save you hundreds of calories per meal by significantly reducing the quantity of oil you are using.

Misters or cooking sprays can be used to flavor foods and to create a nonstick surface for sautéing, grilling, baking, or any form of cooking. Use olive or canola oil to fill your mister—even though both have calories, they're low in saturated fat and, therefore, better for your heart. You can also fill your mister or a spray bottle with salad dressing to keep the calories down. Keep it handy on the kitchen counter so that you're more likely to reach for it instead of the bottle of oil.

Expect to pay $10 to $20 for a good mister (e.g., Misto Sprayer), which you can find in any cookware or department store. If you'd rather use a ready-made version like Pam, keep in mind that although it appears to be calorie-free, a one-second spray contains about seven calories—but you would need about seventeen seconds to equal one tablespoon of oil—so you're still better off.

Steamer Basket:

Steaming is a terrific way to keep calories low without losing valuable nutrients. You can steam chicken, fish, or vegetables—they're all delicious. For about $15 or so, you can pick up a stainless-steel steamer basket, which you insert in a pot of boiling water—it's quick (you only need a small amount of boiling water to create steam), efficient, and easy to use. For extra flavor, add other liquids (e.g., lemon

---

juice, wine, soy sauce, flavored vinegar) to the water, or add your fa-vorite spices (e.g., thyme, rosemary, garlic). Or you can get an electric vegetable and rice steamer, which is a good investment. The Turbo Convection Steamer made by Cuisinart (which costs about $70) has a two-tier design that allows you to steam two different foods at the same time.

Nonstick Pans:

Everyone should have a variety of nonstick pans to help cut down on fat without sacrificing flavor. With a nonstick skillet and a quick blast of cooking spray, you have a recipe for success at any meal—from vegetable and meat dishes to stir-fries and pasta sauces or even egg white omelets. Use just a quick blast of cooking spray, or cook with low-sodium chicken broth or white wine for additional flavor and mois-ture without added fat.

A good nonstick frying pan (like Calphalon) will cost about $30 or so. Keep in mind that you will need to replace your pan as soon as it looks worn out. These pans don't last forever, but you can prolong their life by using plastic rather than metal utensils. Metal scratches the sur-face, and it's essential to keep the nonstick surface intact or you will find yourself using more and more oil to get the job done.

Air Popper:

Instead of making a batch of popcorn on the stove or buying mi-crowave popcorn, invest in an air popper and a bag of kernels. You'll get more popcorn for less money—and you'll save plenty of calories and fat grams. Air-popped popcorn has about thirty calories per cup—not a bad treat. Or as an alternative, NordicWare makes a microwave-safe container you can use to pop *your own* less expensive version of microwave popcorn (about $9). Just take the raw kernels, put them in this dish, and you have microwave popcorn without the expense and, even more importantly, without all the added oils and butter.

Rotisserie Ovens:

You can use these ovens to cook chicken, turkey, ribs, Cornish hens, kebabs—just about anything that you can grill. The concept of a rotisserie oven is to cook food without added fat. You save on calories and maintain the great, natural taste of the food. Or, if you don't want to spend so much money, try a roasting rack that suspends the meat above the pan. For extra flavor, season the meat with your favorite spices, such as rosemary or tarragon, before roasting.

Indoor Grills:

Indoor grills allow you to enjoy grilled foods when outdoor grilling is just not possible. They are usually compact enough to store on a table or countertop right in your kitchen. They use electric burners to provide smokeless, even heat, and offer a nonstick surface that is much easier to clean than a standard, outdoor grill. And best of all, they are designed to drain away unnecessary fat and grease through special sloping grooves on the grilling surface.

One of the most famous indoor grills on the market is the George Foreman Grill, which starts at about $20. Alternatively, opt for one of the nonstick grills that sit on your stovetop and are designed to drip excess fat off the cooking surface into a pan filled with water. Le Creuset grill pans cost about $60 each, and the more affordable Chefmaster stovetop grills run about $15 to $20.

Kitchen Scale:

How much are you eating? It's anyone's guess. Most people underestimate their portion sizes, which is why savvy dieters are using kitchen scales—they're not just for cost-conscious restaurant chefs. Salter makes a variety of models that typically sell for about $50 to $100, but less expensive scales are available, too. There are also scales that give you the nutrient information electronically—right on the scale—so you don't even have to look it up. Measuring cups, spoons, and ladles are also critical tools for the conscientious eater. These are inexpensive and make it much easier to keep track of your portions.

Gravy Separator:

Gravy is often the best part of the dish—but it's full of fattening grease. For about $15 you can purchase a gravy separator (such as the one by Sur La Table). This neat little device looks like something that belongs in a laboratory rather than a kitchen—and it actually separates the fat from the other juices when you're pouring gravy from it.

Prepare Food in Advance

Cheryl never thought of herself as a "stress" eater. Sure, like many of us, when she had a rough day, she would find herself turning to "comfort foods"—those foods that provide a psychological boost or calming effect and tend to be high in calories and fat. But, when she started to audit her behavior and her food consumption, she noticed that she had been eating a lot more "comfort food" than she had thought. In fact, she realized that whenever she had a tough day or situation, the first thought that came to her mind was, "I'm getting myself something good to eat. I deserve a break, and boy, have I earned it."

The problem is that Cheryl's lifestyle was so pressured that, sadly, the importance of comfort food had been blown out of proportion. She works as an attorney, has two teenage daughters, and a husband, who, she says, "is going through a hard time himself, and isn't there for me lately." If you're like Cheryl, you can easily end up consuming a couple of hundred extra calories that you feel you deserve every day, and those calories add up. It seems like only a few bites of a candy bar or half a small bag of chips here and there, so it can't hurt, right? Wrong. A couple of hundred calories per day is 1,400 additional calories per week or almost twenty pounds a year.

When she faced the reality of how comfort foods sabotaged her weight-loss efforts, Cheryl came up with alternative strategies for "treating" herself after a hard day. She began by *thinking before she ate*. She decided to prepare lower fat/calorie dinners *in advance* so that all she had to do was reheat them when she got home. That way, the food would be ready and she wouldn't be tempted to unwind with a candy bar or a cheese Danish as an "appetizer" before dinner.

If you don't like to cook, that's okay, too. It just means you have to keep "quick" prepared foods ready to go in your home. Keeping a supply of healthy frozen foods on hand means that you won't have to think about portion size, which is exactly why prepackaged food plans like Jenny Craig are so successful.

In order to make healthy frozen foods work as 200- to 300-calorie meals you have to make an effort to go to the supermarket and hunt them out. And watch the sodium levels—frozen foods tend to be high in salt. Look for the word *healthy* on the package. By federal law, any foods that say *healthy* (including the brand Healthy Choice) must meet certain government standards: They must contain less than 3 grams of fat per 100 grams and no more than 30 percent of calories from fat. In addition, sodium content cannot exceed 600 mg. Weight Watchers Smart Ones also conform to Weight Watcher's guidelines and cannot contain more than 300 calories or 9 grams of fat per serving.

It's really not so difficult to find the ones that will work for you; just take an extra half-hour or so the next time you go to the supermarket to check out the frozen-food section. Your research will benefit you in the end, and that half hour will translate to several hours saved during the week. Frozen foods are fast, convenient, and many times cheaper than those offered by commercial programs (in addition to which you can pick them up during your regular shopping, and there's no program to join). In fact, George Blackburn, MD, PhD, professor of nutrition at Harvard University School of Medicine, has reported that these types of prepackaged, structured meals (including the ones in your supermarket freezer) are great for long-term, sustainable, weight management. And a study done by Sandra M. Hannum, MS, RD, at the University of Illinois, Urbana-Champaign found that using prepackaged meals was a surprisingly simple way to help study participants lose weight for good.

On your first visit to the frozen-foods aisle, look at labels. Pick a variety of meals that appeal to your taste palate and that provide a portion that will satisfy and fill you. If a frozen meal tastes great, but you need three of them to appease your appetite, it's not the one for you. The choices are endless—from Indian to Italian, Mexican to vegetarian, and chicken to beef platters—all of which can add a little spice into your daily diet. Healthy Choice offers seventy-six dinner and entrée selections, Smart Ones has about fifty-five, and Lean Cuisine has eighty-eight. And the low-carb line Life Choice features fourteen varieties with no more than 15 grams of carbs per entrée. You just have to decide which ones you think you'll like best and can see yourself eating in the long run. For an initial investment of about $50, you can taste test about twenty different meals.

Think about it this way. If you were to get a cheeseburger, fries, and a soda at a fast-food restaurant, that would add up to about 1,500 calories and take at least fifteen minutes with travel, ordering, and waiting time. Frozen dinners, on the other hand, are ready to eat in about four to eight minutes if you heat them in a microwave—and you don't even have to leave your house. Plus, with the calories you'll save (at a minimum you could save 300 calories or more per meal, you're not *always* going to eat out at a fast-food restaurant, and if you do you'll be saving about 1200 calories per meal), if you simply substitute frozen dinners for five of your twenty-one weekly meals, you could cut out at least 1,500 calories per week. Translation: You could lose twenty pounds in one year!

Here are just a few examples that are very low in calories and make great lunches and dinners. I've tried all of them myself, so I know they taste good—at least to me. Plus, I've received plenty of feedback from clients and readers to know that there are ones that *you* will find tasty.

▸ Smart Ones Fajita Chicken Supreme (9.25 oz): 260 calories, 7 g fat, 33 g carbs, 3 g fiber, 18 g protein, 650 mg sodium

▸ Healthy Choice Beef Merlot (10 oz): 240 calories, 8 g fat, 25 g carbs, 6 g fiber, 16 g protein, 600 mg sodium

▸ Lean Cuisine's Chicken Chow Mein (9 oz): 230 calories, 3.5 g fat, 35 g carbs, 2 g fiber, 14 g protein, 670 mg sodium

▸ Life Choice Chicken Parmesan (12.35 oz): 330 calories, 13 g fat, 13 g carbs, 2 g fiber, 38 g protein, 1,110 mg sodium (high in sodium)

▸ Lean Cuisine Dinnertime Selections Grilled Chicken and Penne Pasta (14 oz): 340 calories, 6 g fat, 46 g carbs, 5 g fiber, 25 g protein, 680 mg sodium

▸ Healthy Choice Grilled Chicken Marinara (10 oz): 270 calories, 4.5 g fat, 35 g carbs, 5 g fiber, 22 g protein, 580 mg sodium

▸ Lean Cuisine Café Classics Bowl Chicken Fried Rice (12 oz): 410 calories, 8 g fat, 64 g carbs, 4 g fiber, 20 g protein, 890 mg sodium

▸ Weight Watchers Smart Ones Fire-Grilled Chicken and Vegetables (10 oz): 280 calories, 3.5 g fat, 45 g carbs, 2 g fiber, 18 g protein, 700 mg sodium

▸ Michelina's Lean Gourmet Garden Bistro Asian Style (9 oz): 180 calories, 6 g fat, 29 g carbs, 5 g fiber, 5 g protein, 590 mg sodium

To increase your nutrient consumption without adding many calories and to feel more satisfied, add some frozen vegetables or salad to the meal and cut up a piece of fruit for dessert. And, by all means, put your frozen dinner on a real plate. "The volume of food fills it up, making your portion appear larger, and as a result you will be more satisfied," suggests Hannum. And, in addition, frozen dinners can help you develop a more realistic sense of portion size. "When you're familiar with the size of a 300-calorie entrée, certainly the next time you go out to dinner, or even when you're eating at home, you'll have a better idea of how much you should be eating," says Susan Bowerman, MS, RD, coordinator for the UCLA Center for Human Nutrition in Los Angeles, California.

Since a study conducted by General Mills' Consumer Research Services showed that 80 percent of us make our decisions about what to eat for dinner on the day we'll be eating it, and 40 percent of us don't decide until just before we begin to prepare it, wouldn't it be a good idea to keep these "instant" meals on hand so that we don't make the "wrong" choices at the last minute?

Rethink the Glasses and Dishes You Use

According to a study published in the *Journal of the American Medical Association,* the portion sizes of many foods served in the home (including bread, cereal, cookies, pasta, soft drinks, and beer) have increased by as much as 16 percent. What should you do?

Believe it or not, when it comes to dishes, size matters. Experts have demonstrated that the smaller your plates, cups, or bowls, the less food you are likely to consume. You're more likely to put more food on your plate if it's big, just to fill it. I've seen this in my own kitchen. I used to have oversized bowls that probably held about four cups of cereal. I replaced them with bowls that hold just about one cup and, of course, cut back on my cereal consumption. Clearly this wasn't an act of great willpower—I still filled and finished the bowl. But let's remember: The bowl was *full,* which meant that even if I had wanted to add more cereal, I couldn't! So, let me repeat what I mentioned in the last Step: It's a good idea to measure the amount your plates and bowls hold so that you'll automatically know your portion sizes.

And glassware makes a difference, too. An article published in the *Journal of Consumer Research* by Brian Wansink, PhD, indicates that people who help themselves pour as much as 20 percent more liquid into a short, wide glass than into a tall, narrow one (and teenagers pour as much as 75 percent more). If you keep your glasses tall and narrow, you'll be more likely to keep them half full.

In fact, researchers at Huddinge University Hospital, in Stockholm,

Sweden, reported in *Obesity Research* that vision is one of a number of factors influencing the amount of food consumed during a meal. People ate 24 percent less food when blindfolded without feeling less full. The lesson here is that you need to "fool the eye" to make yourself think you're eating more than you really are.

No More Nighttime Noshing

If dinner is over but you find yourself back in the kitchen, figure out why and what you can do to avoid overeating.

Are you really hungry?

Don't reach into the fridge before asking yourself if you *really* do feel hungry.

If yes

You probably didn't get enough calories during the day, so choose a light snack to satisfy your hunger. But remember, it's a snack, not a second dinner. Small portions of low-calorie foods will satisfy your desire to snack without leaving you feeling overstuffed and guilt ridden. Keep a variety of fresh fruits on hand. Fruit is a sweet treat that doesn't pack on the calories. An apple, orange, or peach has good nutritional value and fewer than one hundred calories.

If no

Put on your diet-detective hat and get to the bottom of your desire to eat. Are you tired, bored, lonely, or just snacking out of habit? If you're tired, go to bed. If you're bored, tackle a project or read a book. If you're feeling kind of lonely and blue, call a friend. Or if it's just a hard habit to break, keep reading for some helpful suggestions to get your mind off food.

Stay busy

Boredom is often the reason for evening snacking, so plan activities to keep you busy. Learn to play a musical instrument, write letters, clean your house, paint your nails, surf the Internet, play with your kids, take a bath, or read a good book. Or choose to do something active after dinner, such as taking a walk, going for a bike ride, or signing up for

---

tennis lessons. After all you've accomplished, you'll feel great and probably won't want to snack any more.

Set snacking guidelines

Here are some suggestions:

- ▸ Eat only at the kitchen or dining room table. Consider all other areas of your home snack-free zones.

- ▸ No snacking in front of the TV (leads to mindless eating).

- ▸ No munching while on the phone (leads to mindless eating and can be really annoying to the person you're talking to).

Serve all snacks on plates. No picking while standing in front of the fridge and no digging into the half gallon of ice cream with a spoon. If you are going to have some ice cream, it must be scooped into a dish first!

Close the kitchen

Once dinner is over, wash the dishes and turn off the lights. Consider the kitchen closed for the night. This may be a good enough deterrent to keep your mind off food.

Drink up

Keep a big glass of water, diet soda, or unsweetened iced tea on hand. Liquid can fill you up, which may subdue your urges to surf the cabinets for late-night munchies.

Remove temptation

Don't keep food in the house that may be hard to resist in the evening hours. Stock your fridge with healthy snacks, such as veggies and fruit, that won't leave you feeling guilty.

Brush your teeth

Once dinner is over, brush and floss your teeth. Food may not be not as tempting if you have minty, fresh breath. Plus, the thought of having to repeat the whole process may be enough to discourage you from eating again. *I offer this suggestion because some of my clients have told me that this works for them, but I do realize that it may not be a strong enough incentive to keep a really powerful craving at bay.*

Keep Foods Out of Sight

Brian Wansink, at the University of Illinois, gave one group of office workers bowls filled with thirty Hershey's Kisses to put right on their desks. He gave a second group bowls that were about six feet away—only three steps. In addition, he used two kinds of bowls—some were clear and some were opaque. What happened?

The people who had the clear bowls right on their desk ate about nine chocolates per day. If the bowl was opaque they ate only about six and a half on average. But, get this, when the bowls were six feet away, whether they were clear or opaque, people ate only four per day. So, where you place your food and how you package it really does matter.

Eat Breakfast

I know you've probably heard this before—no doubt from your grandparents and your parents!—but the research confirms that eating a good breakfast every morning is critical to losing and maintaining weight. In fact, research reported by the University of Colorado says that 78 percent of successful weight-loss maintainers were found to eat breakfast every day of the week. Make sure your personal environment is set up so that you eat breakfast every day. But what does a "good" breakfast consist of? In a study done taking a large sampling of the United States from 1988 to 1994 and reported by the *Journal of the American College of Nutrition,* the researchers found that eating cereal (either ready-to-eat or cooked) or quick breads for breakfast is associated with significantly lower body-mass index than either skipping breakfast or eating meats and/or eggs. Cereals and breads are typically lower in fat and higher in fiber than eggs and/or meats—and as for skipping breakfast altogether, that will only ensure that you're hungrier when lunch rolls around (or by the middle of the morning). Cereal is quick and easy to prepare. Just be sure the ones you choose are low in sugar, and watch your portion size.

Keep This in Mind

According to a study completed by Yunsheng Ma, PhD, MPH, and reported in the *American Journal of Epidemiology:*

▶ If you eat at restaurants for breakfast or dinner you are twice as likely to gain weight because restaurant foods are usually higher in calories and fat, have lower fiber, and their big portions encourage overeating

▶ People who skip breakfast are 4.5 times more likely to be overweight

▶ Eating four or more meals a day reduces your chances of being overweight by 45 percent.

Create an Environment for Social Support

I used to think that asking for support was really just asking people you know to act like the "food police"—watching your every move to make sure you stuck to your diet—although that never seemed to work for me. If someone in my family told me not to eat something, I just took it as all the more reason to show my independence and shove that croissant down in two defiant bites. Then I felt doubly bad. Guilty for eating the croissant, and ashamed for disappointing both myself and my family.

In actuality, however, social support means the opposite. It's having your family, friends, and/or community facilitate your helping *yourself* to lose weight.

Essentially, there are two types of group support. Research has shown that we can benefit either from participating in an organized social support group (i.e., self-help groups such as meetings at churches, community halls, or even commercial weight-loss centers), or by having the support of family and friends.

In fact, the city of Philadelphia is a great example of how providing social support led to weight loss for participating citizens. About three years ago, Mayor John Street set up a health and fitness initiative in response to Philadelphia's being named "America's Fattest City" by *Men's Fitness* magazine.

Philadelphia's "Health and Fitness Czar," Gwen Foster, MPH, created "Fun, Fit, and Free," a citywide program focusing on group support as its primary mission. Her concept, "We are all stronger, smarter, and richer than one of us," was the driving force behind the program. With the backing of Mayor Street (who at one time weighed in at 300 pounds), Foster's office set up more than 200 social-support group centers in hospitals, churches, synagogues, and even at City Hall. According to Foster, the average participant successfully lost 5.3 pounds in twelve months.

Timothy Patton, RD, MPH, professor of public health at Florida International University, also reports that support from a community can provide many psychosocial advantages including:

▸ Emotional sharing: It provides a shoulder to lean on and an ear to listen.

▸ Empowerment, encouragement, and motivation: A group is more than just the sum of its parts—one plus one equals three. Group members can be more successful together than any of them would be on their own.

▸ Mentoring, problem solving, and coaching: It helps to talk to people who have been through a similar experience.

▸ Networking and sharing of information: People in a support system can tell each other about the latest and greatest information— a new diet book, a healthy recipe, etc. This is one of the primary reasons why groups like Weight Watchers work for so many people.

And what about support from family and friends?

Well, imagine trying to lose weight while your husband, wife, family, or friends are constantly urging you to eat fattening things. They might try to convince you, "It's okay to eat that—it's your birthday, anniversary, the weekend (or any excuse)."

Or perhaps they keep telling you, "You're fine just the way you are," and "you don't need to lose weight." Your so-called support group may not want to see you suffer through yet another diet. They may even be trying to sabotage your efforts because they are jealous of your newfound goals, or because they feel guilty about not having made the same choice to pursue a healthier lifestyle.

On the other hand, study after study has shown that solid family and social networks can positively influence your health. It's not a leap of faith, therefore, to infer that strong support from family and friends brings an increase in self-confidence by validating your choice to lose weight, a reduction in overall stress, and increased attention to achieving your overall goal.

In fact, having a weight-loss buddy can help you to win your battle of the bulge. A study by Rena R. Wing, PhD, professor of psychiatry and human behavior at Brown University, found that friends who followed a weight-loss program together lost more weight and were more likely to complete their diet program and maintain their weight loss than those who were going it on their own.

Among those in the study who dieted alone, 76 percent completed their program and 24 percent maintained their weight loss during the 4- to 10-month study period. However, of the group that dieted with the social support of friends (which included group cooperation as well as having team competition between other groups in the program), 95 percent completed their program and 66 percent maintained their weight loss in full.

So, what should you do to improve your social network for maximum weight loss?

Get Organized: Look for organized meetings in your area that discuss and share weight-loss issues. See if your community has any type of organized event. If not, maybe you should start one.

Get Them to Join In: Try to encourage your friends and family to eat healthier without being a nag. Come up with creative ideas, possibly even having different "weight-loss teams" competing for some big prize for the group that loses the most weight. If you can manage to change your social environment—meaning get your spouse, family, and friends to change their habits—it can have a positive impact on your health-related behavior. Think about it—if you didn't have bags of cookies lying around the house, fast-food meals being waved in front of you, or large-scale Italian dinners tempting you to forget your newfound healthy behaviors—oh, how much easier it would be to shed those unwanted pounds.

Pitch In: If you're not the primary food preparer in your household, offer to help out with shopping for healthier foods and planning lower-calorie menus.

Make New Friends: Try to find your own weight-loss buddy at a gym, community organization, or church group, someone in a similar situation who is also attempting to lose weight. Or look for Web sites that offer secure buddy boards—there are many organized, quality, message boards with free group support.

The Company Counts: Eating with family, friends, coworkers—it all adds up. Eating with family and friends can be a real diet buster. So, if your friends and family are poor eaters and don't exercise (or if they seem to be able to eat anything they want without gaining a pound), be prepared.

I'm not saying you can't be social or involved with these people, but you do need to think about your behaviors and plan in advance. Step 9 will provide you with additional skills for learning to mentally prepare for these situations.

It also wouldn't hurt to make a few new friends who are health and fitness conscious. *Mind you, I'm not saying replace your old friends*—just find a few new ones who don't carry that extra Hershey bar in their briefcase or purse. A critical factor in your potential for successful weight loss is the company you keep—that is, the people within your social environment.

Keep the Family Peace: Sit down with your family and have a reasoned, rational discussion about why it's critical for you to lose weight. Explain that they don't have to modify their way of life, but they should at least support your objective. Just make sure it's clear you don't want them watching all your food choices like a hawk. I don't know about your family, but that could start an all-out war in mine.

Parties and Social Occasions: If you're eating at a friend's house, you don't want to make your host uncomfortable by offering up explanations of why you aren't eating his/her food. But there are a couple of things you can do to improve the chance of there being something on the menu you can eat. You might be generous and bring a low calorie, low-fat dessert or side dish such as a fruit salad or vegetable plate. Your host will no doubt see this as a gracious gesture, and you will have avoided a potential food disaster. Or, you might call your host in advance and let him/her know that you're on a medically restricted diet. The term "medically restricted" is usually all you need to say to receive a positive response and avoid too many questions.

On the Job

Policemen get doughnuts. Executives get catered lunches. Even Santa gets cookies. Nearly all jobs present some sort of challenge to people who are trying to follow a healthy eating plan. Does your job entice you with tempting, high-calorie goodies? Do your well-meaning coworkers bring in chocolate or trays of home-baked brownies? If so, there are a few things you can make automatic in order to prevent their good intentions from finding their way to your waistline.

Career Fare: The "Un-Health" Benefits

Declare a No-Food Zone: Set up a neutral territory where unhealthy food cannot be left for others. The zone might be no bigger than your desk, but at least that's a start. And who knows? Perhaps others who are also watching their weight will take a cue from you.

Do Not Leave Candy on Your Desk or in Your Drawers: You will eat more candy—or any food for that matter—the closer it is to you.

Buddy Up: There's strength in numbers! Team up with a coworker who is also trying to make healthy food choices. The two of you can serve as emotional support and reminders for each other.

Veg Out: Wash and cut fresh veggies the night before, or buy them ready-to-eat from your supermarket or local deli. Pull them out for a quick munch when others are snacking on salty, high-fat chips. You'll feel much better about yourself for making the healthier choice!

Water It Down: Keep a full water bottle at your desk and sip it at regular intervals. Not only will you be well-hydrated, but water will help keep you feeling full without adding calories.

Pack Rat: Plan your meals in advance and pack them to go the night before work. Don't forget plastic cutlery if necessary! Pack snacks to eat at regular intervals during your workday. They'll keep you from getting too hungry between meals. The hungrier you are, the more likely you'll lose control and make an unhealthy choice.

Catered to You: If clients or sales reps like to provide catered meals on occasion, ask to be told in advance when this is going to occur. Try to find out what will be served and if healthy choices will be available. Scope out the scene, checking for heavy dressing on salads, mayo in the sandwiches, creamy sauces on the entrées, and extra cheese on the pizza. Load up on the veggies and steer clear of the desserts, opting for fruits instead.

Chew on This: Sugarless gum is an excellent way to keep your mouth busy without adding inches to your waistline!

Breathe Easy: Freshen your breath and leave a clean, minty feeling in your mouth by brushing your teeth after your meals at work. This can help cut down on your desire to munch on high-fat sweets. Invest in a spare toothbrush, paste, and holder to keep in your desk.

Single It Out: If you are going to indulge in a sugary treat, serve yourself one portion, take it to your desk, and eat it there. Do *not* start eating directly from the bag, pan, or serving plate. If you do, it will be difficult to keep track of how much you are eating.

Do Your Duty: You were hired to work, not to eat. Concentrate on completing the tasks you were assigned instead of taste-testing all your coworkers' homemade cookies. Direct all that energy and focus toward a larger salary instead of a larger waistline!

Eat Out and Lose Weight

When you're at home, it's slightly easier to have a healthy stock of vegetables on hand and to limit the quantity of fattening foods in your personal environment, but the farther you get from home, the harder it is to control your environment, and this is particularly true when you're dining in a restaurant. Those are the times when you really need to *think before you eat.* The FDA is now advocating that restaurants be required by law to disclose the nutritional content of their food (something that fast-food restaurants are already doing), but until a new law is passed, when you're eating out, it's still a matter of buyer beware. Therefore, the better laid your plans are in advance, the more likely it is that you'll *automatically* make the best choices.

I love going out to dinner—the starched tablecloths, uniformed waiters, top-notch service, the whole atmosphere—I get hungry just thinking about it. Let's face it: Eating out is entertainment. In fact, the National Restaurant Association estimates that we eat almost six meals per week outside the home (about 290 times per year)—which means that if you overeat by 200 calories each time (an extra couple of pats of butter), you're looking at an extra 16.5 pounds per year. The problem is that we go out to eat and want it to be a special occasion, but something as simple as *not* putting sour cream on your baked potato or skipping that extra piece of bread can go a long way toward preventing your overdoing it.

Plan Ahead: You will learn more about this in Step 8, The Power of Planning, but for now, try these important tips.

▶ Call the restaurant ahead of time to find out if healthier options are available, and/or check out the Web site. You can probably even place a special order in advance. There's almost no restaurant that doesn't have some kind of grilled chicken, fish, or lean meat, a vegetable, and a salad.

▶ Dine at an earlier or later time; restaurants are more likely to be receptive to special instructions during off-peak dining hours.

▶ Make your choices before you sit down. Never go to a restaurant without preplanning what you're going to eat. You may think this would take some of the fun out of restaurant-eating, but a large part of the experience of eating out is being with friends and loved ones and enjoying the good conversation. So, try it. It may just work for you. And if you don't want to plan your whole meal in advance, try developing a selective perception: Train yourself to only see the foods you know you should be eating. Just choosing among salads, fish, lean meats, and poultry will afford enough (but not too much) variety, and after a short while, you'll barely notice the gnocchi.

▶ Stay away from buffets and all-you-can-eat restaurants.

▶ Avoid the price-fixed menu that encourages you to eat more than you need or want.

Be aware that it's harder to make the right choices when dining out with a group of friends—try to focus on choosing well, and don't feel forced to order an appetizer just because everyone else is.

Don't Eat Just to Eat: For many of us, devouring the bread basket is a way to fill the time, not just our stomachs, until the real meal comes. To avoid being tempted, and if your fellow diners agree, ask the waitperson not to bring bread to the table. Or, if you must have a slice of bread, at least don't smother it with butter or dip it in olive oil.

▶ French bread (four slices): 384 calories, 4 g fat, 72 g carbs

▶ Garlic bread (four slices): 545 calories, 21 g fat, 75 g carbs

▶ Butter (two pats): 72 calories, 8 g fat, 0 g carbs

▶ Olive oil (2 tablespoons): 240 calories, 27 g fat, 0 g carbs

Snacking on peanuts or other bar treats to pass the time while waiting for your dining companions to arrive just adds calories to your dining-out experience.

▶ Peanuts (¼ cup): 212 calories, 18 g fat, 7 g carbs

▶ Tortilla chips (1 cup): 130 calories, 7 g fat, 16 g carbs

▶ Pretzels (1 cup): 171 calories, 2 g fat, 36 g carbs

Eat Before: Avoid going out to eat when you're starving. Have a high-fiber snack beforehand, like an apple or even a bowl of cereal. And don't skip meals before eating out because you think you'll save calories; the hungrier you are, the more you will eat. Try calorie-free liquids like seltzer, diet soda, or herbal teas before your meal—they will fill your stomach up.

Avoid Large Portions: According to a survey by the American Institute of Cancer Research (AICR), 69 percent of Americans say they finish their entrées all or most of the time. If you know that the restaurant you're going to serves huge portions, don't assume that you won't eat everything you're served. Just ask the server to wrap up half your portion in a takeout box.

Skip the Pasta and the Fries: If you think you're going to have just one or a couple of bites and leave the rest, well, you're mistaken. Just say no—to the side of fries or pasta, that is. Replace it with a healthy portion of broccoli steamed with garlic or some other type of vegetable or salad.

▶ French Fries (one medium order): 450 calories, 22 g fat, 57 g carbs

▶ Pasta with meat sauce (1 cup): 301 calories, 10 g fat, 33 g carbs

Don't Be Afraid to Ask: Don't refrain from asking your waitperson questions or making special requests because you're embarrassed. You are the only one who will suffer. I often tell the server I'm allergic to certain foods (just to make it simpler). And remember that if you didn't like a food—say the gorgonzola on a Cobb salad—you would have no problem speaking up and asking your server to leave it off, so don't be embarrassed in this situation either. Remember, restaurants want you to be satisfied because your business is important to them—so don't be shy. Ask how your dish is prepared even if it's called *light* on the menu.

Also, make sure to ask:

"Is this dish fried?"

"Can you make this dish without frying?"

"Can you steam the vegetables/fish?"

"What is the sauce made with?"

"Can you prepare this without the cheese/sauce?"

"Can you put the sauce on the side?"

"How large is the serving?"

"How many ounces is the beef/chicken/fish?"

"Can you make this dish without soy sauce/MSG?"

Read the Menu: Look for any of the following: baked, grilled, broiled, poached, or steamed. These cooking techniques use less fat and are generally lower in calories. Avoid any of the following words: à la mode (with ice cream on the side), au gratin (covered with cheese), battered, bisque (made with milk or cream), breaded, buttered, cheese sauce, creamy or rich, crispy, deep-fried, deluxe, fried, hollandaise (sauce made of butter, egg yolks, and wine), jumbo, nuts, scalloped, sautéed (unless you make a special request for it to be prepared in a small amount of oil), and tempura. Be conscious of "selling" menus. Don't be tempted by the words on the menu, they're designed to entice you, and be wary of the dessert tray—prepare in advance. And if everyone is having dessert, simply plan to join in the experience by having a latte or a cappuccino made with skim milk while your dining companions have their cake (but only if it's comfortable). Or if you need to go further, and you must have something sweet, try ordering a plate of fruit or berries. The main point is to think about these kinds of situations in advance and know how you're going to handle them—that way you won't be caught off guard, and behaviors like these will become automatic in the future.

On the Side: Ask for dressing, sauces, butter, or sour cream on the side instead of on the dish itself. If you dip your fork into the dressing and then take a bite of salad, you'll be eating a lot less dressing than if it was tossed with the salad in the kitchen.

Salad Sabotage

Here are the calorie, fat, and carbohydrate counts for 3 tablespoons (a standard restaurant serving) of a few popular salad dressings.

▸ Blue cheese: 231 calories, 24 g fat, 3 g carbs
▸ Caesar: 233 calories, 25 g fat, 2 g carbs
▸ Ranch: 222 calories, 23 g fat, 2 g carbs
▸ Thousand Island: 177 calories, 17 g fat, 2 g carbs
▸ Creamy Italian: 150 calories, 15 g fat, 3 g carbs
▸ Olive oil and vinegar: 210 calories, 23 g fat, 1 g carbs

Liquid Doughnuts: Don't go overboard on the alcohol—it adds excess calories, stimulates your appetite, and tends to encourage you to forget whatever plans for healthy eating you made in advance. If you want a drink, have it with your meal rather than before.

If you're trying to lose or control your weight, watching your alcohol consumption can be essential. Simply having one beer a night adds up to more than 1,000 calories per week—that's an extra fifteen pounds per year. And a couple of glasses of wine over the course of a meal can easily add as many as 400 calories. It's the alcohol itself that contains most of the calories, so it's time to forget the idea that by having *hard* alcohol you'll be keeping the calories down while getting more buzz for your buck. There are seven calories per gram of alcohol, compared to four calories per gram for either carbohydrates or protein. So the lower the alcohol content of the drink, the fewer the calories.

▸ Dry table wine (8 oz): 165 calories, 0 g fat, 3 g carbs
▸ Beer (12 oz): 148 calories, 0 g fat, 13 g carbs
▸ Margarita in a pint glass: 676 calories, 0 g fat, 43 g carbs

And remember, nonalcoholic beverages (soda, juice, sweetened iced tea) also add calories. Just two or three sodas add up to about 400 calories!

Fast-Food Help

Simone French, PhD, a professor of public health at the University of Minnesota, reports that eating just three meals per week at a fast-food restaurant was "associated with increases in body weight, total energy intake, percentage fat intake, intake of hamburgers, French fries and soft drinks, and with decreases in physical activity, dietary restraint, and low-fat eating behaviors."

Know What You Are Going to Order in Advance: Almost every fast-food restaurant has their nutrition information on the Web or at the restaurant. Find out what's available ahead of time. Plan what you can have in five or six fast-food places and you will never be forced to decide on the spot and overindulge. By doing that you'll be making your choices second nature.

Drink to Your Health: Drink plenty of water, orange juice, or skim milk instead of soda. This will boost the vitamin and mineral content of your meal.

Toss the Sauce: Eliminate condiments, relishes, toppings, special sauces, dressings, and garnishes because they are high in fat, sodium, and calories.

Sub That Grub: Substitute mustard for mayonnaise.

Beware of Portion Distortion: Practice portion control and resist the urge to super size.

Get Fruity: Carry a couple of pieces of fresh fruit (e.g., apples), or take along carrot sticks or sliced red bell pepper and enjoy them with your meal instead of fries. You'll be getting the crunch without the fat and calories.

Way to Go, Tomato: Instead of sauce, give your sandwich a healthy, juicy taste by adding tomatoes (which are fat free and packed with immune-building vitamin C).

Blot a Lot: Cut down on the fat by blotting your French fries, pizza slice, or hamburger meat with a napkin before you eat them. Blotting your pizza can save as many as eighty fat calories!

Don't Be Cheesy: Instead of cheese, opt for lettuce, tomato, and onion; taking off one slice of cheese will subtract about one hundred calories.

Veg Out: Top your pizza with vegetables instead of meat and cheese.

Toss Out Your Hunger: Order a tossed salad and enjoy it before the main meal to curb your appetite.

Go the Extra Mile: Ask for extra veggies with your stuffed pita sandwiches.

Dare to Share: Share a sandwich with a friend (but make sure the sandwich is a healthy one).

The Snack Attack

We all love to snack. Whether it's in front of the TV, in the office, at the café with your morning coffee, or simply as a mid-afternoon treat, a snack can get you through the good times and the bad. But snacking, as we've already discussed, has also been associated with adding extra pounds. A survey conducted by the Calorie Control Council has revealed that 33 percent of adults list "snacking too much" as a reason for being unsuccessful at losing weight. It's therefore pretty safe to assume that you, too, will be experiencing snack attacks. To ensure that you stick with the program at those tempting times, try to implement the strategies I suggest for making sure that you *automatically* go for the kinds of snacks that will satisfy without sabotaging you.

It Doesn't Make You Fat: The Centre for Food Research at Queen Margaret College in Scotland reports that snacking does not necessarily predispose people to becoming overweight. In fact, those individuals who snack throughout the day may actually have the advantage over those who conform to a rigid pattern of three meals a day because well-balanced snacks keep hunger in check between meals, so you're not starving by the time dinner rolls around. The key, however, is choosing the right foods to snack on.

Late Dinner? Eat Protein: If you're planning a late dinner and need a snack to tide you over, choose something with additional protein, like a few nuts, a piece of low-fat cheese, or low-fat yogurt. The scientific journal *Appetite* reports that consumption of a high-protein snack delayed the request for dinner by sixty minutes—much longer than either a high-fat (twenty-five-minute delay) or high-carbohydrate snack (thirty-four-minute delay).

Avoid Carbs—Have Mini-Meals: According to Jackie Berning, PhD, RD, nutrition professor at the University of Colorado, a food that contains primarily carbs (e.g., fat-free pretzels) does not make a good snack because it will digest in about two hours. Instead, Berning recommends having "a mini-meal, such as five or six crackers with string cheese," which would take longer to digest.

Be Prepared: Just as with regular meals, you should have healthy snacks available when you want them. Come up with five different low-calorie snacks you enjoy and keep them on hand at all times. "You should create snacks that are about 100 to 200 calories, depending on your daily calorie needs," advises Berning.

Eat More: Since portion control is very often a struggle, it's critical to pick snacks that are low in calories so that you *can* eat more if you *need* to overindulge. Try low-calorie, low-sugar, and high-fiber cereal that you can eat dry (e.g., Kashi)—it's great to munch on and can help you avoid putting on pounds. As a rule of thumb, assume you are going to eat as much as 50 percent more than you think you will.

Keep Your Home Safe: Most snacking is actually done in the home—all the more reason to keep high-calorie snacks out of your house and out of sight. If you have a snack attack, and there isn't any bad stuff around, you're more likely to automatically go for the good stuff. Or perhaps it won't tempt you—then the craving will pass, and you'll be grateful.

Afternoon Guard: Again, don't worry so much about the morning. According to the *Journal of the American Dietetic Association,* afternoon is the most common time for snacking. So in the afternoon, make sure you have low-calorie snacks—such as soy chips or fat-free yogurt—within reach.

The TV Adds Pounds: The scientific journal *Eating Behavior* reports that watching TV induces high-calorie snacking. Results suggest that snacking (but not necessarily eating meals) while watching TV is associated with increased overall caloric intake, as well as increased calories from fat.

At the Movies? Many theaters have a "don't ask, don't tell" policy when it comes to bringing in healthy snacks—meaning they're not checking your bags and policing the aisles looking for your baggie of chopped up celery sticks. Bring in foods that don't smell and won't get crushed when they're shoved into your bag. Focus on foods that are nutrient dense—that is, filling and low in calories—so that you can munch on them mindlessly throughout the movie, just like popcorn.

Since we're probably not really paying attention to the taste anyway, I wonder how many of us would know the difference if our movie popcorn was replaced by Kashi cereal, Cheerios, or even a bag of cut up vegetables? See if you notice. Also try:

▸ Homemade air-popped popcorn—at only 30 calories per cup, it's a good deal

▸ Beef jerky—especially if you're an Atkins fan. (It's salty, so try to find the low-sodium versions.)

▸ Fruit—apples are not easily crushed when hidden in your bag. It's a good idea to cut them into slices

▸ Rice cakes—watch the calorie and fat content

▸ Energy bars—a bit better than those king-size chocolate bars

---

Snack Intelligence

Here's a list of tasty snacks to help you make smarter choices next time you're grabbing a quick bite on the road or at the local coffee house:

With Your Coffee

Worst
Starbucks Classic Coffee Cake (139 g): 570 calories, 28 g fat, 75 g carbs, 7 g protein

Bad
Dunkin' Donuts Maple Walnut Scone (one scone): 470 calories, 22 g fat, 62 g carbs, 6 g protein

Middle of the Road
   Dunkin' Donuts Glazed Cake Donut (one donut): 350 calories, 19 g
   fat, 41 g carbs, 4 g protein

Almost Healthy
   Au Bon Pain Low-Fat Triple Berry Muffin (123 g): 290 calories, 2 g
   fat, 61 g carbs, 5 g protein

Nutrition Savvy
   Starbucks Chocolate Hazelnut Biscotti (28 g): 110 calories, 5 g fat,
   15 g carbs, 2 g protein

Chocolate Craving

Worst
   Fried Snickers with Powdered Sugar (one bar): 598 calories, 43 g
   fat, 48 g carbs, 6 g protein

Bad
   Fudge (85 g): 392 calories, 16 g fat, 58 g carbs, 4 g protein

Middle of the Road
   Balance Gold Triple Chocolate Chaos Bar (50 g): 200 calories, 6 g
   fat, 22 g carbs, 15 g protein

Almost Healthy
   Kudos Chocolate Chip Granola Bar (one bar): 130 calories, 5 g fat,
   20 g carbs, 1 g protein

Nutrition Savvy
   Swiss Miss Diet Hot Chocolate with Calcium (one packet): 25 calories, 0 g fat, 4 g carbs, 2 g protein

Savory Snacks

Worst
   Cheddar Cheese Pretzel Combos (one single-serving bag): 240
   calories, 8 g fat, 35 g carbs, 5 g protein

Bad
   Terra Chips (one bag—42 g): 220 calories, 11 g fat (2 g saturated
   fat), 27 g carbs, 2 g protein

Middle of the Road
   Baked Potato Chips (one bag—60.2 g): 220 calories, 3 g fat (no saturated or trans fat), 46 g carbs, 4 g protein

Almost Healthy
   Glenny's Barbecue Soy Chips (one bag—36 g): 140 calories, 3 g fat,
   18 g carbs, 9 g protein

Nutrition Savvy
   Air-popped Popcorn (3 cups): 92 calories, 1 g fat, 19 g carbs, 3 g
   protein

Don't Be a Diet Hero

Avoid cues that are going to tempt you. If you drive by a Dunkin'
Donuts on the way to work every day and you know you'll be tempted to
stop, change your route. Stay out of the supermarket when you're starving. Don't leave foods in the house that are going to set you off. Ask
your family for their cooperation. When it comes to losing or maintaining your weight, as with most things in life, there's no point in asking
for trouble.

Get Out There and Explore

The more of these tools and strategies you have in place, the better
able you'll be to replace your old negative patterns with new, automatic,
healthier patterns. Now it's time for you to get out there and start
exploring—your own food preferences; the possibilities for small compromises; the nutrient labels on the foods you've been eating and those
you might want to substitute; the Calorie Bargains waiting to be discovered in your supermarket; ways to safeguard your personal food environment; and new choices to be had in restaurants. It's a big world out
there, and now that you've learned how to safeguard your environment,
you should be able to seek out new possibilities you probably weren't
even aware of before. Automating your environment shouldn't feel limiting; it should be the key to your feeling empowered to enjoy all the
world has to offer.

Discover Your Fat Pattern: Be a Diet Detective

"I believe that one of the characteristics of the human race—possibly the one that is primarily responsible for its course of evolution—is that it has grown by creatively responding to failure." —Glen Seaborg

"Quitting smoking is easy. I've done it a thousand times."
—Mark Twain

You have now begun to build the foundation for creating a Livable Diet and making it automatic for the rest of your life. At this point it might be tempting for you to think: "I've got it—find my Calorie Bargains, make the substitutions, watch out for a few food traps, and make it all routine." My answer to that statement is yes, you do have it, but only part of it. In order to make this *automatic*, to make it stick, you still have six more critical Steps. Stopping here would be like planning a vacation and saving enough to buy airline tickets and pay for a hotel room, but not having any money to see the sights or buy food.

In the following Steps I'll be teaching you how to do the investigative detective work that will allow you to bring your fat patterns out into the open by looking at your Individual Dieting Traits (IDTs), and then giving you practical advice *you can use right now* to cope with Unconscious Eating, your Eating Alarm Times, and those Diet Buster situations and occasions when you're most likely to fall off your diet. Discovering your fat patterns and identifying your Diet Traps are steps toward new ways of thinking. And if you don't learn to think differently about what you've done in the past, you may find your *diet* history repeating itself.

Like anything in life, when it comes to our relationship with food, we can—and should—learn from experience. And sometimes bad experiences can be our best teachers. As William Saroyan, internationally renowned writer and playwright, has said, "Good people are good because they've come to wisdom through failure."

So, how does that bit of wisdom translate into daily life? Let's say you wake up and wander into the kitchen early one morning. Sleepily, you put your hand down to reach for the handle of the coffee pot. Unfortunately, on this particular morning, your spouse has already made the coffee and left the pot off-center on the burner so that the handle has been heating up over the very low flame. When you touch it, you're shocked by searing pain! What do you do next?

Thrust your burning hand under a stream of cold water? Get angry with your spouse for being so careless? There are many possibilities, but here's one thing I'll bet you won't do: You probably *won't* reach out for that steaming-hot coffee pot the next morning without using a bit of caution, like grabbing a pot holder. You got burned once, and that was enough.

But if bad experiences can be such good teachers, the key question we need to answer is, "Why do we sometimes make the *same* dieting mistakes over and over again? Especially when we've been burned by so many diets and promises?"

One reason is that, in truth, changing our "fat" patterns is not as simple as learning from a scalding hot coffee pot; unfortunately, these patterns run deep, and they can be quite insidious. Oh yes, they may be right out there in the open for you to see, but you can still be blind to them unless you make a conscious effort to "see" them. It would be great if our eating patterns burned like the hot, coffee pot—then maybe we wouldn't be so quick to grab at them again. But they don't.

What we need to do, therefore, is to take a long, hard look at what we've done in the past so that we don't get burned again. The *Annals of Behavioral Medicine* has reported that "historical factors including an individual's previous dieting attempts and their weight history" do play a role in current dieting success. In other words, by examining our "fat" patterns, we can learn what we *should* and *should not* to do to make our eating *livable, automatic, sensible, effective,* and *satisfying* in the future. You're going to learn to do that—you've just experienced your last "burn" with the diet you just finished.

Learning from the Past to See Your Future

So how can looking at your past help you?

Any fat pattern you may have, whether it's eating candy, snacking late at night, not exercising, or mindless eating in front of the TV—whatever it might be—provides you with some kind of emotional/psychological benefit (e.g., reduces stress, entertains). This is important to keep in mind because, as we delve a bit into your past, it will help you to remember that *you shouldn't be too hard on yourself for being the way you are*—there is a reason you have been doing what you're doing. It's not because you're weak or have no willpower, *it's because you have been receiving a benefit from your current patterns.* The benefit is that the eating makes you feel better, fills you up, comforts you, and provides you with fuel—the problem begins when you overconsume. Now, I'm not going to tell you that you need to examine every last detail of your life in order to find out how to lose weight. But, I will ask you to go through a series of written exercises that have been "time-tested" by my clients over the years, and that really help to shed light on your unique eating pattern.

The great thing is that you are the creator of all your own food preferences—your individual attitudes and feelings about food, your automatic eating responses, your use of comfort foods during times of stress—basically, what food means to you at the deepest level—which means you are in a very unique position:

You have the power to change them.

If you understand what you are doing (such as making excuses for why you should eat another half-box of cookies), and why you are doing it (you had a fight with your best friend), you have a better chance of being able to break the "cookies-as-comfort-food" pattern. A careful and honest examination of past successes and failures allows you to see the outline and substance of very distinct patterns. By recognizing these patterns, you can analyze them, see why and how they occurred, break them down, and focus on stopping the destructive behaviors—ending the vicious cycle of the diet. You also learn to turn things around and capitalize on your *positive patterns. You can harness these positive patterns to make huge advances and lose weight for good simply by making a conscious effort.*

The operative word here is *conscious.* Click into your consciousness and out of unconscious patterns, and then create a *new,* more positive pattern of eating and physical activity—one you can live with comfortably—one that fits you just right.

Be kind to yourself and tell the truth about what, when, where, how, and why you eat the way you eat. Once you identify your negative eating patterns, they can be broken and replaced with *healthier* automatic ones that will eventually be just as simple to follow as your old patterns.

How Did We Get These Fat Patterns Anyway?

Mental-health researchers tell us that we establish patterns of behavior early in life, and the way we eat is one of those behaviors. According to the scientific journal *Nutrition Review*, parents provide a child's contextual environment for weight-related problems.

Rachel is the perfect example of how that occurs. Every time Rachel was upset as a child she was given sweets to calm her down. While this is not the *sole* reason for her current behavior, she continuously seeks sugary food to comfort herself during emotional times. Rachel learned early on that sugar can reduce stress and calm her during an otherwise difficult, emotional situation.

Unfortunately, Rachel's pattern of eating for comfort has led to her being significantly overweight.

In essence, Rachel has the benefit of reduced stress from high-calorie, sugary foods, but the consequences are now causing her emotional and physical discomfort. I'm sure Rachel knows that being significantly overweight is worse than feeling occasionally sad or stressed. But at the moment she goes for the sugar, she's simply not thinking about the long-term effects on her weight—she's not standing there thinking, "Oh, if I eat this it's going to go right to my hips." She might even make a statement to that effect, but she is really not being conscious of what she's saying or truly connecting her statement to the effects of her consumption. Her behavior has, over time, become a pattern.

But why would Rachel continue to eat for comfort even though it doesn't help her to reach her long-term goal of losing weight and getting in shape?

The trouble is that there are many, many variables that stop us from behaving the way we say we would *like* to behave in terms of eating and physical activity. One of the strongest influences, suggests Judith Ouellette, PhD, a professor of psychology at SUNY Cortland, is that it's how we have always behaved in the past when a particular set of circumstances arose. We may think that eating a box of cookies led to our being overweight, but the fact that eating cookies is what we have always done when we were in a stressful situation causes it to seem like what we should continue to do. In other words, it works, we've always done it, we don't see the connection to anything negative, so why stop. Throughout our lives, habitual patterns form the strongest basis for predicting behavior in the future.

And the primary reason Rachel continues to do what she's always done is that she doesn't know how to apply other available, more positive strategies for feeling comforted.

If Rachel is ever to triumph over her emotional eating pattern, she won't do it by exerting superhuman willpower over wanting that extra cookie, but by realizing that her eating pattern isn't working in her best interest and coming up with other, effective ways to find comfort during stressful times. How can she do that? By becoming a "diet detective" and honestly seeking out the facts and rituals that have led to her weight problems.

Being a Diet Detective

To start the process of identifying patterns that no longer work for you, you have to delve into your history. This delving is *not* so you can find people, circumstances, or events to *blame* for your food patterns, but to help you see what does and doesn't work.

The idea is to be a diet detective in your own life—except that in this case you are not only the detective—you're also the culprit!

Detectives do a number of things. For instance, if a detective were looking into a burglary at the local bank, the first thing he or she would probably do would be to review the scene of the crime and attempt to identify some of the potential perpetrators by looking into their prior bad behaviors and past experiences. Detectives look for any clue that might lead them to a conclusion. They interview people who know the suspect, and they begin piecing together the psychological and physical evidence to come up with some sort of illuminating profile.

These are the same concepts you should apply when you're identifying and reviewing your dieting patterns. Look back, seize on the relevant details, and let them help you prepare for a resolution—in your case, creating a livable, effective diet you can take with you throughout your life.

Combining self-reflection and self-assessment leads to awareness. And awareness is one of the tools you will use to overcome the factors of genetics, hormones, and all the other influences that are making it difficult to reach your desired weight and body shape.

To guide you in your investigation, I've put together a list of some of the "usual suspects"—questions, details, and solutions with regard to some of the common dieting behavior I've seen in dealing with clients.

▸ First, we'll look at your dieting history.

▸ Then, we'll run through the lineup of Individual Dieting Traits, IDTs, that I see again and again in my search for negative dieting patterns. You'll be able to pick your own IDTs out of the lineup.

▸ Then, in the following Step, we'll continue the detective work by identifying and helping you to overcome your Diet Traps—those behaviors and influences that repeatedly get you into diet difficulty.

Your Dieting History: The Good, the Bad, the Diet

Since "those who do not learn from history are doomed to repeat it," this is your chance to change history and finally win the battle of the diet wars. The *American Journal of Clinical Nutrition* reports that nearly 91 percent of "successful losers" had previously failed in their efforts to lose weight. Many reported losing and regaining the weight—up to nearly 270 pounds—before they finally mastered permanent weight loss. Even 70 percent of those who had been overweight from childhood were ultimately able to succeed.

Not only that, but what I've learned from my clients is that the ones who maintain their weight loss are those who *took a look back—not to find fault or blame with past diets—but to see what they could learn!*

With that in mind, I want you to think about the weight loss and exercise strategies you've tried in the past—those that worked and the strategies that didn't. The purpose of this activity is to do a little housecleaning—get rid of the stuff that doesn't work and use only the stuff that does.

Keep in mind, when looking at your past, that it's not unusual to camouflage certain unpleasant or unflattering details or truths about yourself. Everyone does it.

An honest and uninhibited look at your history is a courageous and potentially healing act that will ultimately change your future for the better. By embarking on a voyage of self-discovery with an open heart and mind, you can expect to have an "Aha!" experience—that moment when you finally see things as they really are and identify the underlying structure that governs your behavior and personality.

To start, list three strategies that worked when you've tried to lose weight in the past. For each strategy, write down why it worked for you.

For example, you might write: *I love hardboiled eggs, so I would always have them prepared, peeled, and ready in the fridge for when I had a snack attack. I didn't mind having egg snacks. It worked for me.*

Or:

I was in Weight Watchers, so I had a support group. The members of my group really cared about my success. They helped me to learn that it was okay to want support. I'm for whatever works so I can lose the weight.

Or:

When someone first suggested keeping a food diary, I thought, "You have to be kidding." Well, I was the one kidding myself. I had no idea that keeping a diary even for a couple of days could be helpful. I purchased a tiny notebook and wrote down every detail of what I ate. I figured out the calories, fat, carbs—and I was amazed. I was eating much more than I had ever thought. It really surprised me.

Now it's your turn. In your notebook, write down the *three* diet and activity strategies that worked for you in the past.

1 . . . 2 . . . 3 . . .

Now list five strategies that *have not* worked when you've tried to lose weight in the past. This will probably be much simpler than having to come up with the strategies that worked! Make sure to include a detailed description of why you believe these strategies didn't work and what you have learned from them. Here are just a few examples of unsuccessful strategies that come up again and again with my clients.

All the dieting gurus told me, "don't deprive yourself." Well, I didn't deprive myself all right. Whenever I had a desire for cookies, I would eat them. I would try having just one, but I simply couldn't stop myself. I put on ten pounds following the "don't deprive yourself diet."

Or:

Doing any kind of physical activity in the morning was a disaster for me. I would set three alarm clocks, have my gym bag ready, but no matter what, sleeping was more important than a half-hour jogging around the park.

Or:

Eating a low-carb diet was great in the beginning, but I found myself missing bread, pasta, and other good foods. I thought I could last forever on that kind of diet, but it just didn't work. I regained all the weight I'd lost after a year.

Now, write down the *five* dieting strategies that haven't worked for you.
1 . . . 2 . . . 3 . . . 4 . . . 5 . . .

Okay, now what? You wrote down the strategies that have and haven't worked. How is that going to help you lose weight? Research on the subject of weight control and dieting has shown that all these past efforts do count—no matter what the outcome. In fact, the more you try to lose weight and fail, the greater the chance of succeeding the next time. I know what you're thinking: "If failing is the key to winning the diet war, I should be in perfect shape right now." But it's not quite that simple. You also have to *do something* with the information you've just collected about yourself in order to *break the pattern* of previous disappointments.

You can learn from every diet you're on, but the key question is: Can you use what you've learned to make changes that will work in your life, and for the rest of your life? Your past attempts to lose weight were not wasted.

For instance, I've had clients who discovered that they didn't need two slices of bread to feel satisfied by a sandwich—just the meat and veggies, wrapped sandwich-style in a lettuce leaf are satisfying on their own. And I know clients on Weight Watchers who learned to make sure they surrounded themselves with people who were supportive of their efforts and new lifestyle. And finally, clients who worked with Jenny Craig have learned portion control by eating the foods, and nutrition education from the one-on-one counseling provided by the program.

So now, take all the things you've written down and go through them carefully. Think about them and hold on to the facts, the attitudes, and the behaviors. You'll need to remember what worked and what didn't so that you can use the good stuff and not repeat the bad.

Continuing the Investigation and Identifying Your Individual Dieting Traits (IDTs)

Just as we have preferences for particular styles of entertainment and activities such as movies or sports, so will we choose the *dieting style* we think suits us best. In the case of diets, however, whatever style we choose, it typically ends up disappointing us in the end.

Now that you've looked to your own dieting history for clues, I'm going to introduce you to a cast of characters that, as a diet detective, I run into again and again when investigating diet patterns. These are the habitual behaviors, which I call Individual Dieting Traits (IDTs), that create individual "fat" patterns.

As I describe these characters, chances are that you'll recognize yourself in one or more of them and that they'll provide you with insight into some of the behaviors you may have missed in the course of your own dieting career. Many times clients think they know exactly what's been preventing them from moving forward, but the reality is they just don't see it. They need a bit of a nudge, which comes in the form of examples of other people's experiences.

Read them with your notepad at hand and pick out the traits you identify with in your own dieting lifestyle. Do you snack unconsciously? Do you consider foods offered by others at the office or social events "free," and therefore not part of your calorie intake for the day? Once you have the most complete dieting profile you are able to compile, you'll be able to view your past dieting behavior through a new lens and see where you went wrong—or right.

Seeing yourself in others is one way to gain some of the information you'll need to solve the mystery of how you can control your weight. It's also encouraging and comforting to know that there are others who have dealt successfully with issues that are similar to your own. You might say, "Well, they were stronger and had more willpower." But I'm here to tell you that even though we are all different and need to approach our situations individually, you can learn from other people's dieting failures and successes. So keep an open and observing mind and read on.

The Diet Food "Expert"

Sam, a thirty-eight-year-old computer technician from South Carolina, was about thirty-five pounds overweight—and an on-and-off-again dieter for the last twenty-five years. He believed he was a diet-food expert who could reach the holy grail of dieting by eating every low-fat or low-sugar food. As long as it was labeled a "diet" food, Sam was okay. In fact, Sam was a *misguided* diet-food expert—he was really just a diet-food junkie.

Sam hadn't lost any weight, but he still had faith in what he believed was right, even as it proved him wrong. The problem? Low-fat foods are typically high in sugar, and low-sugar or low-carb foods are usually high in fat. Sam believed the promises made for all the low-type foods and indulged in all of them to excess. Since he thought he was eating diet food, he ate as much as he wanted without guilt or considering the consequences.

Essentially, people like Sam are always seeking the latest and "newly improved" diet food without understanding what makes up basic, good nutrition. By insisting he was on a diet, Sam didn't take responsibility for his food choices or why he didn't lose weight. Instead, he preferred to live in denial.

Sam was finally able to break his patterns by recognizing that just because something is labeled "diet food" doesn't give you license to overconsume it. When Sam took the Three-Day Food Challenge and tallied up all the calories he was eating, he was shocked. Sam also realized that he—not the manufacturer or the food label—was responsible for his food choices. He became more of an investigator and picked his foods more carefully. He still uses "diet food," but now he uses it to his advantage, not to his detriment.

The Diet Groupie

The Diet Groupie is personified by my client Barbara, who lives in Southern California. Every time I spoke with her, she told me about a new diet she was on to lose the seventy-five extra pounds she'd been carrying since grade school. Barbara enjoyed the idea of being up-to-date on the latest diet. She talked about diets nonstop, bought all the books, followed the newest diet star on the talk-show circuit, and made the diet she happened to be on her religion. At thirty-eight years old, Barbara still got incredibly excited by each new diet as a new sense of hope emerged. And every single time, without fail, she lost weight, only to gain it back as soon as she got bored with the diet and realized that it wasn't the one for her.

Barbara was always looking for the BBD—the Bigger Better Diet—believing that something new and exciting would sweep her off her feet and take her out of dieting hell forever. She would rather try someone else's new program, which she believed would require very little work on her part, than come up with her own diet—one that would really let her lose weight and maintain the loss for life.

Barbara told me that she just couldn't "dwell on" why she jumped from one diet to the next or why she overate, but she did say, "I just want to *lose the weight quickly*. Tell me what to do!" Once Barbara focused her energy on learning how to set herself up with a plan and strategies for achieving her goal, she succeeded for the very first time. The way she kept the weight off was by picking lower calorie, tasty foods—her Calorie Bargains—and using what she'd learned from past diet failures, (i.e., seeking social support, restocking her kitchen) to create a *foolproof* automated environment in her home and her social life. She also learned to take dieting a bit slower, realizing that those who lose weight quickly are also most likely to regain it.

I'll Start Tomorrow Dieters

How many of us have said we're going to start a diet tomorrow, after the weekend, after the holidays, after the summer, after the winter, when we're thirty, forty, fifty, etc.? I'll Start Tomorrow Dieters have the rap down pat: They don't want to start dieting until *after* some momentous upcoming feast or event, like Thanksgiving or a birthday bash. And frequently their calendars are so full that tackling their weight issues is always a long way off. Other events simply take priority.

No matter what the excuse, putting off the inevitable doesn't help. If you want to lose weight, you can start *any time*. And the sooner, the better!

The Unreal Exercise Junkie

Denise, from Chicago, was twenty-seven years old and went to the gym faithfully for about an hour every day. She walked on the treadmill, did a fast circuit, and put in time on the elliptical trainers, but she never lost a pound. Why not? Because Denise used the gym for entertainment, and she deluded herself into thinking she was doing everything she could to lose weight. "My gosh," she moaned, "I'm at the gym *every* single day. Why isn't exercise working for me?"

She blamed bad genes for her love handles and wide hips. Plus, she believed that regular exercise should be enough to take off the pounds: "Isn't that what all the experts claim—an hour a day to lose weight?" The fact is, Denise liked to eat, not exercise.

If you looked at her food diary, you'd see that she ate a pint of frozen yogurt almost every day and paid little attention to her overconsumption of other foods. She'd never even thought about how much she was actually eating. And, although she was at the gym every day, she was really just going through the motions. But even if she'd been maximizing her time at the gym, she would have nullified her effort by eating that pint of frozen yogurt. Going to the fitness center on a regular basis is a good move, but it gave Denise the false impression that her activity level was "extremely active" and she could, therefore, eat as much as she wanted, which was not the reality.

Eventually, Denise was able to recognize that exercising was not a license to overeat, and that her estimate of what she was consuming—or could consume for her activity level—was inaccurate. She began to spend a lot more time planning and coming up with better eating strategies and was able to slowly lose the weight. The fact that she exercised was wonderful and a tremendous advantage for Denise. So as soon as she realized she could still eat foods she liked while being more conscious of her choices, she was able to put together a diet and program of physical activity that worked for her.

Just Too Busy

Barney and Sloane are a married couple who lead a busy life. Both of them work, and they say they have no time to shop for food, much less time to cook or even think about what to feed their two kids. Sloane told me that everyone in her family ate high-sugar cereal for breakfast, then grabbed a deli sandwich, usually ham and cheese or tuna salad with lots of mayo, and a bag of chips or a side of potato salad (also packed with mayonnaise) for lunch. Even her kids, who bought lunch near their school, were going high fat.

After work, she picked up the kids from the sitter, met her husband, and they all had dinner at their favorite, family-style restaurant on the way home. They relaxed over dinner and drinks and discussed what they could stop and pick up to have for a snack or dessert when they got home—usually high sugar or high-fat/salty snacks. The kids tended to go for the chocolaty treats while Barney and Sloane preferred salted nuts or microwave, butter-flavored popcorn.

Since they were Just Too Busy, they were worrying about everything *except* why they were gaining weight. But stopping to shop for nutritious food and snacks doesn't take any more time than shopping for desserts and sugary breakfast cereals. And it would have benefited their entire family to rethink their use of time and what their lack of attention to smart eating was costing them.

Barney and Sloane needed to develop a plan, so I worked with them to come up with quick strategies that fit their hectic lifestyle, such as creating a list of restaurants and takeout places where they knew they could preselect foods that were low in calories but tasty and filling. They also discovered snacks that were healthier, and made sure that they always had a supply in the house. In the end, they lost weight, saved money, and had more time to enjoy each other.

It's Justifiable

People who feel justified are comforting themselves from past stresses or unpleasant events. Samantha was one of those. She came up to me after a lecture I gave not too long ago and asked if I could give her some advice. She was more than 150 pounds overweight, about forty-five years old, and deeply concerned about her weight. She told me that her father had abandoned her and her mother when she was a small child, and she believed she was using food to soothe herself and using her weight to hide from the world. By being overweight she was allowed to disappear. She believed that if she looked unattractive, a factor of her obesity, she could exile herself from the world and be unavailable. She wouldn't exist in the social whirl; she'd never have to face rejection from another man; and she'd never have to be hurt again by someone she loved and trusted.

Consequently, whenever she felt lonely, sad, or bored, which was nearly every day, Samantha used food as medicine for what ailed her. Food was an easily available drug. Although she understood what she was doing to herself, she still couldn't manage to get past the first step: not overconsuming junk foods.

She'd been in counseling to deal with her emotional issues, but hadn't yet been able to move forward with her weight issues, much as she wanted to. Her dilemma was founded on the misconception that her father's abandonment gave her a reason to eat what she wanted, and that it was all justified. To some extent, Samantha was right—she had good reason to feel sad and vulnerable as a result of her childhood experience. But she was ready and wanted to move on and live a full, happy life, not continue to sabotage herself and make excuses for her situation. The point she'd missed, or couldn't emotionally connect to, however, was that being overweight—which her "medicine" was causing—was doing her far more harm than good.

Samantha worked to understand the core concept that you may not be responsible for certain events that took place in your life, but you are responsible for how you react to them and what you do next. She was confused because she felt that life had dealt her a bad hand, which was compounded by her being grossly overweight. It took a number of exchanges before I finally got her to understand—without minimizing her pain—that while certain events had hurt her, they were in the past, and it was now up to her to solve her weight problem and live life, not hide from it.

The Restrictor

Jeff, a restaurateur from Kentucky, complained that he just couldn't seem to lose weight. "I think I must have the slowest metabolism in the world, and I'm not going to starve to death to get fit. There must be some diet that will work!" he'd say. He was on a diet that consisted of nothing but steak, chicken, and cheese—no bread or vegetables or fruits—along with all the fat he could eat. He'd follow this diet to the letter at mealtimes, but since he was still hungry between meals, he'd resort to snacking on whatever food was in front of him, and a lot of it!

Peanuts at the bar, half a pie as an after-dinner treat, a bag of chips when he was out and about. He figured he was still on the diet because he was eating nothing but tons of meat and cheese during his planned meals, yet the unplanned snacks he needed to make up for his hunger were preventing him from losing weight.

I tried to get Jeff to take the traditional Three-Day Food Challenge, but he felt that keeping a food diary even for only three days was too much of a burden. So, we came up with an alternative. We had all the bartenders and wait staff in his restaurant keep track of every single thing he nibbled or ate when he was there. After three days, we examined the results. Needless to say, Jeff was shocked. We then focused our efforts on teaching him about the effect that diet deprivation has on shedding pounds, and how to think about tough food situations in advance so that he would be mentally prepared during his time in the restaurant. The point here is that you need to adopt a method that works for you. Jeff didn't want to keep a food diary, so we improvised— improvising was the theme of his livable diet.

Each of the people described above had a different eating and/or activity pattern. Have you found the one (or ones) that best describe the reasons for your own dieting discontent? It may well be that you fit more than one type. To refine the search and make identifying your patterns even clearer, let's move on to discovering some more of the clues—Understanding Mindless and Unconscious Eating, tracking your Eating Alarm Times (EATs) and learning how to control them, and mastering your Diet Busters.

◀◀ STEP 5 ▶▶

Master Your Diet Traps

"Experience is not what happens to a man, it is what a man does with what happens to him."

—Aldous Huxley

After working with thousands of clients, doing significant research, and working in public health, I've identified the key behavioral issues that are the real diet traps, or potentially self-sabotaging eating habits, and how to manage and stop them. A Diet Trap can be a certain food you can't resist, or a situation and/or event that is either comforted or celebrated by food. Most of all, a Diet Trap weakens your determination to meet your weight-loss goal. Everyone has Diet Traps, but anyone can beat them and get back on track.

Diet Traps can arise from:

▶ Unconscious and Mindless Eating
   Delayed Feeding
   Entertainment for the Mouth
   Social Eating
   Comfort or Stress Eating

▶ Eating Alarm Times

▶ Diet Buster Moments

In this Step, you will learn to identify and begin to manage your Diet Traps and take the next step toward creating a livable, workable diet.

To begin, let's examine the one trait most people tend to overlook: *unconscious eating.*

Unconscious and Mindless Eating

You're sitting in front of your computer, you're tired and bored, and you have a project due at the end of the day. As you're sitting there, you open a drawer and pull out a box of cookies left over from a birthday party the week before. First it's just one cookie. Then it becomes two. Before you know it, the whole box is gone. Sound familiar? You just consumed well over 1,800 calories. Or, perhaps you pick at food all day while doing tasks, but don't really taste what you've eaten after the first bite. You can put away thousands of extra calories a week just like that—by eating without thinking.

This is all about Unconscious Eating, and it manifests itself in two forms. The first is eating in a mindless, automatic way, like finishing the cookies in front of your computer without even realizing it. How many times have you said to yourself, "I was satisfied after the first two. So why was I compelled to eat more? Why couldn't I just stop instead of eating until I felt sick?"

The other type of unconscious eating is consuming food without being aware of the calories you munch. How often do you eat foods without having any idea of their nutrient value—or, more specifically, the number of calories the food will cost you (not in terms of money, but in terms of added weight)? When you have a cup of coffee and a muffin for breakfast, you may not have even a ballpark estimate of how many calories that muffin contains.

Most people wouldn't walk into a store and buy things without knowing the price of what they were buying. So why would you put anything into your mouth without knowing the cost: the calories, carbs, and fat content, especially since most food comes with a tag, called a "food label"? Maybe because you'd rather not know! The problem is that ignorance isn't bliss, and not knowing doesn't save you any pounds. Through *conscious and aware* eating, you actually increase your choices because paying attention to the nutritional breakdown of what you're eating gives you opportunities to look for foods that are satisfying and tasty but relatively *inexpensive*, at least in terms of calories.

Conscious eating means eating when you're hungry, enjoying the taste, smell, and texture of each bite of food, and knowing the food's nutritional content. Unconscious eating, on the other hand, puts you in a kind of fugue or semi-dream state during which your hand automatically dips into a bag of junk food or you just keep opening your mouth and eating a meal without thinking about *how much* until you've eaten a lot more than you intended. It involves eating without paying attention to the experience. For example, standing in front of the refrigerator picking at a leftover piece of cheesecake while talking on the phone is mindless. And interestingly, in your estimation, these random bites probably don't even really count toward your day's total calories.

There are many reasons why people eat mindlessly, but Delayed Feeding, Entertaining the Mouth, Social Eating, and Comfort or Stress Eating tend to be the most popular.

Delayed Feeding

You skip breakfast because you're on the run, and you're really not *that* hungry. Or, you could really go for something but don't have the time, or your kitchen cabinets and fridge are bare. Before you know it, 2 PM has rolled around and you've had nothing but a few cups of coffee and maybe a buttered roll. You're primed to eat the first thing that crosses your path. Typically, in that situation you don't sit down and think of what would be healthy. Your body is telling you you're hungry, you're preoccupied with your work (or your kids), and there it is in the distance—a box of chocolate-chip cookies. A coworker or friend comes over holding out the open box. Then he or she actually leaves the box on your desk, and you indulge. You take three, scarfing them down so fast your mind doesn't even register that you've eaten. In any case, your mind is on your work, and you're staring at your computer trying to finish that report you've been focused on for days. Before you know it, you've downed six cookies. That was almost 500 calories you didn't even realize you'd eaten. Not only that, but the food you just ate is not nutrient dense, and the calories are not going to satisfy your hunger, so you will eat more.

How often have you been on the go and not eaten for a long while? As soon as you see a coffee shop, deli, or a fast-food restaurant, everything on the menu looks delicious, so you eat and *overeat* because you are hungry. What about food shopping on an empty stomach? Avoid it. Shop on a full stomach or else you will end up buying all the "wrong" unhealthy foods, and probably tearing open up a bag of chips while you're waiting in the check-out line. Most people either wait too long between meals or skip meals and wait until they're ravenous and willing to eat anything. Unfortunately, at these times, the tendency is to choose foods that are high in calories and fat. Delayed feeding can be treacherous to your waistline, especially if you skip breakfast.

It is generally agreed, and an article in *Obesity Research* has confirmed, that eating breakfast is a characteristic common to those who maintain successful long-term weight loss and may be a factor in their success.

So, don't skip this meal.

Entertainment for the Mouth

Watching TV is entertainment for the brain and the eyes. Unfortunately, TV, movies, and computers don't entertain our mouths and stomachs, so we eat to entertain them, and sometimes we engage in both forms of entertainment simultaneously.

Take TV viewing, for instance. *Eating Behavior* has reported a revealing study on how people snack in front of the TV. Not surprisingly, the researchers concluded that the TV is a *stimulus for eating. What* is eaten during these times was significant: In one study, researchers concluded that people will eat *snack foods rather than meals* while watching TV, accounting for an increased overall caloric intake and too many calories from fat.

The same would be true for the movies. I can't tell you how many times I've been at the movies, engrossed in the film, munching on a bucket of popcorn and a box of candy, when, all of a sudden, I put my hand in the popcorn container and there's nothing left. I could have been chewing on the *New York Times* and it would have been the same. It was a waste because I wasn't paying attention to the popcorn, so I didn't even enjoy it.

I'm not alone in the popcorn sweepstakes of mindless consumption. Believe it or not, popcorn consumption is the worthy subject of many studies, including one done by Professor Brian Wansink and a team of researchers at The Food and Brand Lab at the University of Illinois who asked the question: Do external cues, like attractive packaging and perceived good taste, impact how much of a product you'll consume? Using stale movie theater popcorn as bait, the answer they got was "Yes," with a capital Y.

Here's when excess calories sneak in for you and me. The study found that moviegoers who rated the popcorn as tasting relatively *unfavorable* ate *61 percent more* of what they *didn't like* if they were given a large container. One reason, say the researchers, was that consumers find it more difficult to monitor how much they're eating *from a large container*. And I'll add the other factor: At the movies, your focus is going to be on the screen, so you click into mindlessness gear and eat whatever is at your fingertips.

When you're focused on one thing or multitasking, avoid shoveling high-calorie, high-fat, high-carb food into your face. The truth is, it's just not worth it.

Social Eating

You're sitting at a restaurant, having a great conversation with family or friends, and the bread basket is on the table along with an excellent bottle of red wine. You're enjoying yourself. You eat a few pieces of bread, dip it in oil, and have a couple of glasses of wine. You're having fun, eating, and socializing, and, for the time being, you're oblivious to what you're consuming—or perhaps you've just let yourself off the hook, figuring, why not, you only live once.

Another scenario: You get to a party and your hosts are serving appetizers. You may not even be hungry, but you eat because the food is right in front of you. You're probably not even aware that you're eating. Or you help yourself to a few brownies just because someone brought a few trays to the office. It's there, it's free, and so you go for it.

I went to a discount supermarket recently and was amazed by the long line of people waiting for a free sample of a new brownie mix. People were waiting almost twenty minutes for a one-inch chunk of brownie—not even a sample of the mix to take home and whip up! It was also a spontaneous social occasion, with strangers chatting about brownies—their favorites, how to make them, and so on—and looking forward to having a taste when they got to the head of the line.

Clearly, the idea that "it doesn't count because it's free" is a very real problem, and one that many would-be dieters have made their mantra. It's time to chant another tune, so to speak. "The human body is an amazingly fine-tuned machine, which is one of the reasons that eating a few bites here and there—fifty to one hundred calories—can add on extra pounds over time," says Rachel K. Johnson, PhD, MPH, RD, a professor of nutrition at the University of Vermont. *"Just a bite"* truly counts.

The way to solve the problem is *don't edit your eating!* In the *beginning* of this process it's important that you keep track of what you're nibbling when cooking, cleaning up, eating off other people's plates, dipping into samples at the grocery store, munching idly on nuts or pretzels at a bar, or even grabbing a Hershey's Kiss from the communal bowl at the office so that your awareness itself will become automatic, and soon you'll just know what to do without thinking about it. Here are a few suggestions to avoid the "nibble" factor:

▸ Stay conscious of your "picking times," that is, when you're most likely to pick at food.

▸ Stay away from key "picking areas," such as the kitchen or a buffet table.

▸ Avoid leaving candy dishes or bowls of chips and other foods out and within easy reach.

▸ Skip free samples at stores, and don't feel you have to pick from other people's plates because you don't like "wasting" food.

▸ Curb your urge to take a sip of someone else's beer or soda or to take a few swallows from the juice container when you open the door of the fridge.

Social eating is another form of entertaining your mouth. You eat because it's there, and this time it's the party or other social event that's the entertainment, not the TV or a movie. Food is what we use to fit in and to keep ourselves entertained, or to calm social anxiety, or just to seem polite.

How Much Can Those Little Nibbles Here and There Add Up To?

Passing Through the Kitchen

▸ Four tablespoons Häagen-Dazs Butter Pecan Ice Cream: 155 calories, 11.5 g fat, 10.5 g carbs

▸ Five Lay's Classic Potato Chips: 40 calories, 2.5 g fat, 3.75 g carbs

- One Oreo Double Stuf cookie: 70 calories, 3.5 g fat, 9.5 g carbs
- Ten Rold Gold Classic Tiny Twists Pretzels: 65 calories, 0.6 g fat, 14 g carbs
- A handful of Quaker 100% Natural Cereal (granola) with oats, honey, and raisins: 109 calories, 3.5 g fat, 18 g carbs
- A handful of Cheerios: 28 calories, 0.5 g fat, 11 g carbs
- A handful of trail mix: 174 calories, 11 g fat, 17 g carbs
- One Hershey's Kiss from the candy bowl at work: 25 calories, 1.5 g fat, 3 g carbs
- A handful of raisins: 86 calories, 0 g fat, 23 g carbs

Eating While Out and About

- A slice of brie cheese: 189 calories, 16 g fat, 0 g carbs
- Four wheat crackers: 76 calories, 3 g fat, 10 g carbs
- Two heaping handfuls of movie theater popcorn: 168 calories, 13.5 g fat, 9 g carbs
- One bite of a hot dog at the ball game: 48 calories, 3 g fat, 4 g carbs

While Cooking or Cleaning

- Crumbs at the bottom of a bag of Pepperidge Farm Nantucket Double Chocolate Chunk Cookies: 140 calories, 7 g fat, 18 g carbs
- The slices/edges of pie or cake that are trimmed before putting it away so that it looks neat and even: 86 calories, 5 g fat, 9 g carbs
- A spoonful of Pillsbury Chocolate Chip Cookie Dough while making cookies: 32 calories, 1 g fat, 5 g carbs
- One spoon of just the chocolate chips: 80 calories, 4 g fat, 10 g carbs
- Peanut butter on a knife while making a sandwich: 95 calories, 8 g fat, 3.5 g carbs
- Whipped cream off the beaters: 52 calories, 5 g fats, 1 g carbs

Eating Off Someone Else's Plate

- Two forkfuls of chocolate cake that you would never order—but will gladly eat when someone else does the ordering: 117 calories, 5 g fat, 17 g carbs
- Leftovers from your kid's Happy Meal at McDonald's: 10 fries:

53 calories, 2.5 g fat, 6.5 g carbs; 2 bites of a McDonald's cheeseburger: 80 calories, 3 g fat, 9 g carbs

Leftovers

- ▶ Two bites of cold Pizza Hut Hand-Tossed Cheese Pizza: 77 calories, 2 g fat, 11 g carbs
- ▶ Three forkfuls of beef chow mein: 68 calories, 4 g fat, 3 g carbs

Drinks

- ▶ A sip of someone's beer: 24 calories, 0 g fat, 2 g carbs
- ▶ A sip of Tropicana Orange Juice from the carton in the fridge: 28 calories, 0 g fat, 6.5 g carbs
- ▶ A sip of soda: 25 calories, 0 g fat, 7 g carbs

Comfort or Stress Eating

You had a rough day with your children, your car broke down, your boss was angry because you finished a project late, and you have no idea what you're going to make for dinner—you are stressed out. Where can you seek refuge?

How about in a slice of cheesecake, a box of candy, a pint of ice cream, a pizza, a taco special, an order of fries, or a sixty-four-ounce bottle of cola and a bucket of fried chicken? These goodies are always quick to the rescue in our times of need. Over the years we've comforted ourselves by gravitating toward this kind of food, thinking, "I only live once, so I might as well enjoy myself now."

"When tension and anxiety are high in one aspect of life, it's not unusual for other areas to seem trivial or less important," says John Foreyt, PhD, director of behavioral research at Baylor College of Medicine. "This shift in priorities can lead to a breakdown in behaviors that may normally be under control, such as our diet."

There are psychological and biological reasons why we turn to food for comfort. Certain foods are associated with a time in the past that was nurturing or loving—food is a symbol of care giving. And when it comes to body chemistry, these comfort foods can cause the release of brain chemicals, such as endorphins and serotonin, that produce a calming effect. In fact, if you're suffering from a bad day at work, screaming kids, premenstrual syndrome (PMS), seasonal affective disorder (SAD), a fight with family or friends, or even if you're on vacation and just want to chill out, a small dose of carbs might do the trick.

Two renowned scientists, Richard Wurtman, MD and Judith Wurtman, PhD, at the Massachusetts Institute of Technology (MIT) were the first to connect food with mood when they found that carbohydrates boosted a potent brain substance called serotonin. Serotonin is a neurotransmitter that controls mood, sleep, and appetite, and, when elevated, helps you to feel more relaxed and calm.

Here's how it works: The glucose in high-carbohydrate food triggers the release of insulin. This in turn allows the amino acid tryptophan to reach the brain (by blocking other competing amino acids), stimulating the production of serotonin. We need that sense of calm to stop the cycle of stress eating, but *which* foods we choose to help us achieve it can make all the difference between gaining and controlling weight.

Researchers have said that when palatable foods are consumed, the body releases trace amounts of opiates, which elevate both your mood and your sense of satisfaction. Although these opiates are released in small amounts, opiate-related food rewards may reinforce a preference for the foods that are most associated with these feelings.

Comfort Food Favorites

A survey of over 1,000 North Americans conducted by the researchers from the Food and Brand Lab at the University of Illinois at Urbana-Champaign found that America's favorite comfort foods are:

1. Potato chips (23 percent)
2. Ice cream (14 percent)
3. Cookies (12 percent)
4. Chocolate (11 percent)
5. Pizza or pasta (11 percent)
6. Steak/burgers (9 percent)

Comfort foods are an interesting topic because they have such a strong emotional component. Each of us has his or her own version of comfort food—and, believe it or not, it can be a plate of liver and onions for one person as easily as it could be a giant bag of pork rinds for another. There's always an X factor involved with why we choose what we choose.

A University of Illinois study on comfort-food preferences pointed to this psychological motivation. These motivations, it turns out, are usually related to factors such as "social context, social identification and conditioned responses"—all of which influence the development of food perception and comfort-food preferences.

The problem is, when someone is feeling down, he/she tends to go for foods that are not only high in carbohydrates, but are also high in processed sugar and fat. "When people are feeling gloomy, they attempt to self-medicate with food," says Elizabeth Somer, MA, RD, author of *Food & Mood.* "They go to carbohydrates to feel better; unfortunately, they go to the wrong foods for the right reasons."

So what's the big deal about a few extra calories and fat grams? Well, while food can offer comfort during emotional uncertainty, most experts recommend maintaining control over your internal environment despite the fact that external factors may remain unstable. "During stressful times, it's important to maintain some level of control over your life—especially when your external environment is unbalanced. Being able to look inward and feel good about your nutrition and health is critical," says Dr. Foreyt.

That doesn't mean we have to give up on comfort foods altogether, we just need to be prepared. "Individuals who find themselves engaged in excess eating in anticipation of stress must become conscious of their behavior if they hope to moderate it," says Barbara Schneeman, PhD, nutrition professor at the University of California at Davis.

So what should you eat when you need an emotional boost?

Experts advise *not* eating foods like candy or soda to get your dose of carbs because you could end up feeling fatigued and unsatisfied. "You could get the same boost and crawl out of the hole with whole grains, air-popped popcorn, a whole-wheat bagel, potatoes, winter squash, or corn," says Dr. Judith Wurtman. These foods foster those same feelings of relaxation and tranquility without the ensuing sugar crash.

A little preparation can keep both the psychological triggers and the biological responses to stress under control and stop comfort-food binges from ruining our weight-loss efforts. Once an individual understands that he typically consumes high-calorie and high-fat foods while eating unconsciously, he improves his odds of stopping this harmful pattern. Becoming a conscious eater doesn't take the pleasure out of eating, it simply makes you more aware of how you choose food unconsciously and why you overeat.

Start by weaning yourself off high-calorie comfort foods and onto low-calorie alternatives. Here are a few *comfort food alternatives:*

Instead of: Brownies, 2 oz. (227 calories/9 g fat)
Try: Fat-free chocolate pudding, ½ cup (130 calories/0 g fat)
Savings: 97 calories/9 g fat

Instead of: Hot Chocolate with whole milk and whipped cream, 1 cup (280 calories/15 g fat)
Try: Hot chocolate with skim milk, 1 cup (150 calories/1 g fat)
Savings: 130 calories/14 g fat

Instead of: Apple pie, ⅙ of 8" pie (350 calories/14 g fat)
Try: Baked apple, one apple (100 calories/0 g fat)
Savings: 250 calories/14 g fat

Instead of: Doughnut, 1.5 oz (310 calories/19 g fat)
Try: Low-fat muffin, 1.5 oz (160 calories/2 g fat)
Savings: 150 calories/17 g fat

Instead of: Cheese pizza, one medium slice (280 calories/10 g fat)
Try: Pita bread pizza with skim mozzarella (216 calories/3 g fat)
Savings: 64 calories/7 g fat

Instead of: Mashed potatoes with butter and whole milk, 1 cup (320 calories/16 g fat)
Try: Mashed potatoes with low-fat margarine and fat-free butter-milk, 1 cup (240 calories/8 g fat)
Savings: 80 calories/8 g fat

Instead of: Premium ice cream, 1 cup (600 calories/22 g fat)
Try: Low-fat ice cream/frozen yogurt, 1 cup (240 calories/4 g fat)
Savings: 360 calories/18 g fat

Instead of: Spaghetti and meatballs, 3 cups (770 calories/21 g fat)
Try: Spaghetti and turkey meatballs, 3 cups (630 calories/4 g fat)
Savings: 140 calories/17 g fat

Chicken soup: Watch the noodles, rice, or croutons; otherwise, enjoy. Always try to eat consciously in the ways we've already discussed. Always be there and be aware *before* you eat!

▸ Be attentive to *what* you eat and *when*.

▸ Be attentive to *why* you overeat and what triggered it. Once you are, it will become second nature.

This new reality involves assimilating everything you've read so far: Know your Individual Dieting Traits; be willing to change the way you relate to food and dieting; maintain a positive attitude and keep making the effort to change; disconnect from using food as a drug or a weapon; and, most of all, *set up healthier patterns of eating one small step at a time so that they become a part of your automatic eating behavior to replace the behavior that has not worked in your best interest.*

I'm not saying that you should never indulge in sweets or other treats, but when you eat them, you should try to have a smaller portion you can relish—not use the food as a drug. And always stop when you feel satisfied.

These small changes will make a big difference. I know this is true. It's the little things—such as snacking on a big box of candy at the movies or sitting in front of the TV with a bucket of buffalo wings—that seem to trip up most people.

A new reality that helps you lose weight and ushers in good health is stronger, more empowering, and worth the effort.

Solving the Problem of Unconscious Eating

What are your Unconscious Eating patterns? In your notebook, write down *five* different scenarios where you eat without thinking, and what you can do to prevent Unconscious Eating in that particular circumstance.

For example:

Unconscious Eating: *Eating a large box of popcorn at the movies.*

Preparation to avoid Unconscious Eating the next time it occurs: *I will bring (smuggle) low-calorie cereal and apple slices into the theater. That combo would make me happy. Plus, I would probably feel better if I didn't overeat poor-quality food. Or, every other time I go to the movies I will have a large popcorn, and on those days, I will walk to the theater.*

Remember, this is your life, so create a scenario that works for you. You must become your own Diet Connoisseur.

Pinpoint Your Eating Alarm Times (EATs)

Whether it's late-night snacking, midday munchies, or nibbling while preparing dinner, studies have shown that you can easily cut calories just by focusing on your trigger times, or what I call Eating Alarm Times.

I have done research on the subject of EAT by commissioning a survey of more than 400 people who were attempting to lose weight. The results, subsequently published in *Newsweek* magazine, found that more than 97 percent said there was one specific time of day during which they consumed a majority of their high calorie and high-fat foods. What time of day do you typically overeat? Thirty-four percent of respondents reported eating approximately 400 additional calories during prime-time TV hours, from 8 PM to 11 PM. Next in line was the Afternoon Snack Attack, falling between 2 and 5 PM. Twenty-seven percent enjoyed indulging toward the end of the day when they got home from work or right after the kids come home from school or extracurricular activities—they were using food as a sort of a pick-me-up.

On average, the study's respondents said they ate more than 350 additional calories during these EAT. And the results also indicated that the most popular temptations for overindulgence are what have been called "sin foods," which include candies, cakes, cookies, and other sugary/fatty snacks and desserts.

You need to figure out what to do during your own EAT to prevent overindulging on high-calorie and high-fat foods. If you know that you typically overeat while watching TV, for example, you can develop and rehearse a new plan to keep you away from the "bad stuff."

What Time of Day Are You Most Likely to Overeat?

▸ Breakfast Time (5:00 AM–10:00 AM)
▸ Mid-Morning Munchies (9:00 AM–12:00 PM)
▸ Lunch Time (11:00 AM–2:30 PM)
▸ Afternoon Snack Attack (1:00 PM–5:00 PM)
▸ Dinner Time (5:00 PM–8:30 PM)
▸ Prime-Time TV Snacking Hours (7:00 PM–11:00 PM)
▸ Late-Night Munchies (11:00 PM until. . . .)

One good solution would be to prepare a variety of healthy snacks and meals in advance. Another is to make sure to only have the "better" snacks around the house.

You may even decide to get out of the house a few nights a week and take a class where you know you can't eat. Just as these craving times are different for everyone, the antidotes of choice vary as well.

The idea of having one time of day to focus on is pretty good news: It means we can make real and substantial changes by being a lot more careful just during that one period, when we typically overdo it.

Learning your EAT means that you don't have to overhaul your entire life to lose and maintain your weight. This becomes a key strategy in your arsenal of tactics for creating a livable, automatic diet. So think about the one or two hours each day when you consume the majority of your high calorie and high-fat foods.

Keep in mind, 350 calories (the average amount we eat during these times) can add up to more than thirty pounds a year. Preparation is critical to avoid overindulging, so it's crucial to come up with a plan and mentally rehearse that plan—have your alternatives and adjustments ready in advance. I'll be providing a lot more planning strategies in Steps 8 and 9.

Pull out your notebook, take a look at your own EATs, and try this exercise:

My Eating Alarm Time is _____

My plan is to implement the following five *adjustments* and *alternatives* so that I stop consuming high-calorie, high-fat foods at this time:

1.
2.
3.
4.
5.

Diet Busters

You're at McDonald's with your children. You decide to order a coffee, and, of course, your children order hamburgers, chicken nuggets, and fries. They eat half of what they ordered and stop eating. "Are you sure you don't want anymore?" They say they're finished. The coffee really didn't satisfy your hunger; you only had an apple for lunch because you were on the go, so the next thing you know you're finishing off your children's Happy Meals, fries and all.

In addition to EAT—the regular consumption of high-calorie and high-fat foods at specific times of the day—or Unconscious Eating, not being aware that you are consuming foods—there are less predictable but equally problematic situations that can bust your goals. I call these "conscious eating moments," or Diet Busters.

Diet Busters can be either particular foods that have a powerful effect on you or particular situations and events that knock you off track. Your Diet Buster might be the steaming-hot bread basket that's put on the table at your favorite restaurant, or the delicious pastries your boss brings in every couple of days, or it could simply be the nature of your job or family life.

Diet Buster Foods

When you come into contact with certain foods, it's as if you are hypnotically drawn to them. You feel that the only way to overcome your intense desire for them is to rely on sheer willpower. (We'll be talking more about willpower later.) But rest assured: No matter how many times they've seduced you, nacho chips or s'mores do not control your behavior. Junk food does not contain any of the ingredients of Jedi

Mind Tricks. You are the one calling the shots. And, believe it or not, you *can* stay in control when confronted with a Diet Buster food.

I'm sure you can think of at least three foods that seem irresistible to you. Foods that make you weak in the knees. What foods are they? *What qualities make them so tantalizing?* Write them down below and then, using what you've learned so far, come up with an alternative food choice or a way to make your Diet Buster more resistible.

One example might be:

Diet Buster: Whenever I order a hamburger I ask for it without the roll, but then I eat the mound of French fries that always comes with it.

Solution: Next time I'll ask the server to "hold the fries" along with the roll and get a plain baked potato instead. Or, if I'm feeling really virtuous, I'll ask for a salad, dressing on the side, instead of the potato. I'll still have the burger, which is what I really wanted in the first place.

Now it's your turn to record your *three* most dangerous Diet Buster foods and the solutions in your notebook.

Diet Buster Food:
Solution:

Diet Buster Moments

But Diet Busters are also comprised of situations, circumstances, or events in which you lose your center—your commitment to your intended weight-control plans and your dieting goals is weakened. During these Diet Busting Moments, we tend to slip up no matter how much we intended to stick to our diet. And the sad truth is, these little slipups definitely add up to more pounds and increased frustration. These situations can vary from person to person, and can include special events (e.g., weddings, birthdays, holiday parties) and social situations (e.g., parties, eating at restaurants, or even your occupation). Take Scott's case, for instance.

Scott is a thirty-six-year-old father of two who travels about 130 days per year for business. On his trips, he always makes the same eating mistakes at the airport, on the plane, dining out in unfamiliar territory, and at the hotel-room minibar. These were Scott's Diet Busters. Scott felt that when he was traveling "no one was watching," so he was comfortable eating and drinking whatever he wanted. He was also on the go and just "taking whatever food was available at the time." Of course, these minor food indiscretions added up. Scott overconsumed about 280 calories per travel day, which added up to about 36,400 extra calories per year, or an additional ten pounds.

Scott came up with a series of travel tips that worked to diffuse his own personal Diet Buster. He packed a lunch for the plane and snacks for the airport; he called ahead to the hotels where he was staying to find healthy restaurants in advance; and he requested that the minibar be removed or emptied. He also looked for hiking or walking trails in each of his destinations. Scott was able to lose weight by identifying and then working through his major Diet Busters.

On the Road Again

Whether it's visiting relatives, traveling for business, or taking advantage of airline bargains—many of us travel often. It's hard enough to maintain a healthy lifestyle during the course of your familiar, daily routine, but what happens when you disrupt your normal schedule and habits? Here are a few tips to keep you healthy and sane on your next excursion.

Food for Thought: When you're on your home turf, it's easy to find healthy places to eat, but traveling to a new locale makes it more difficult. Call a hotel concierge for a healthy restaurant recommendation, even if you're not staying at that hotel. Or better yet, ask some of the locals for their favorite, healthy eateries. Be prepared to be specific—there are varying degrees of what one might consider "healthy."

Once you have a few possibilities, phone the restaurants and find out what healthy selections they have to offer (e.g., menu items that are baked, grilled, steamed, or broiled). Don't be shy. Even fast-food restaurants have healthy choices these days (take a look at their Web sites for nutrition information on their products).

Get a room that comes with a kitchen if you can. Most come with pots, pans, and other cooking tools. This way, if you can't find any restaurants that suit your tastes or your healthy lifestyle, you can actually make meals for yourself. In fact, there are many hotels such as Marriott's Residence Inn, Extended Stay America, and Homestead Studio Suite Hotels where rooms with kitchens are standard, and they're reasonably priced.

Keep Cool: If I'm staying in a hotel, one of the first things I ask for is a mini-refrigerator. It's a great way to save on expensive hotel meals, and even better, you can purchase healthy foods (cooked chicken breast, fruit, vegetables, yogurt, milk, etc.) at the local supermarket and keep them fresh in your room. While some hotels charge $5–10 per day for this service, many are willing to give you the fridge at no cost, especially if you tell them you have strict dietary needs. Call ahead, ask if they charge, and make sure they reserve one for you. Also, some places will even put a microwave in your room—it doesn't hurt to ask.

Think Ahead: Prepare sandwiches for the plane (or car) the night before you travel. Most airlines have cut back on food service, so you don't want to end up eating five bags of pretzels or, even worse (in terms of calories), peanuts. Also, pack plenty of healthy snacks. Apples are great—after two hours of not having anything in your system, an apple can taste like a Cheesecake Factory Chocolate Chip Cookie-Dough Cheesecake. Other good ideas include yogurt (in an insulated pack to stay cold), individual boxes of healthy cereal, and cut-up vegetables.

And for goodness sake, eat *before* you go to the airport, even if it's early in the morning. Put something in your system—you don't want to be stuck eating junk food while sitting and waiting at the gate. Airport food is not only costly, it's also very high in calories and fat.

Wherever you're going, be sure to pack a water bottle. Traveling can be notoriously dehydrating, leading to a false feeling of hunger, dizziness, headache, or fatigue.

Virtual Fitness: Keeping fit on the road is not easy, but today most hotels (and homes, if you're staying with relatives/friends) have DVD or VHS players. There are plenty of great exercise videos to choose from. Some of them even come with exercise or stretch bands to make for a better workout. A video or DVD is small enough to slip right into your carry-on luggage. If you have other people staying with you in the room, you might feel a bit self-conscious or embarrassed doing an exercise video in front of friends/family, but you must keep your ultimate goal in sight and remember that it is worth it. Or you can simply wait until everyone goes to breakfast and you can join them twenty minutes later.

For a large selection of exercise videos and DVDs, try www.amazon.com or www.collagevideo.com. To avoid boredom and cut costs, join an online DVD movie rental service such as netflix.com that has a large selection of exercise and fitness DVDs.

Pack Your Gym Clothes: Go online and find a gym in the area you'll be visiting. Try the Web site of the International Health, Racquet, and Sportsclub Association (IHRSA): http://healthclubs.com/find.html. They have over six thousand clubs in their search engine. Once you have a gym in mind, always call first and find out if it will accept "walk-in" guests, and ask if there's a fee.

Take a Hike: Going for a walk and exploring are great ways to take a break from your relatives/friends (if you're visiting), see a new area, and fit in some exercise. Many locations have a visitors' bureau that's filled with information about hiking trails, walking tours, even shopping malls—any place where you can stretch your legs and get some exercise. For a bit of a twist, rent a bicycle for your adventure.

Aside from travel, almost any major life-changing event can also prove to be a potent Diet Buster. Here are just a few you might have experienced for yourself.

Those Life Changes That Bust Diets

Moving is stressful on many counts, and if you're overcome by it, well, you may overeat or eat at random times. Whether it's moving out of your parents' house or into a new home after several years of being comfortable in an old residence, preparations for setting up a new abode can cut into breakfast, lunch, and dinnertime. You're so preoccupied with packing or unpacking that you forget to eat lunch. Then, when dinner comes around you make up for having skipped a meal by breezing into the first fast-food joint you see and super-sizing a burger, fries, and soda.

Divorce also has its misery factor. It inflicts stress on relationships not only with former spouses, but also with children. Divorced people who are not used to being alone turn to food as a source of reassurance—and diets are tossed out the door. In addition, statistics tell us that incomes decrease for women of divorce, which adds even more stress.

Starting a new job is also a stressful situation—you're adapting to new rules, a new boss, a new environment, and new coworkers. All these drastic changes can make dieters turn to food as a source of comfort. Candy, cookies, and other junk foods are quick, easy, and readily accessible, but they're also full of empty calories. And then there are also new food sources. Perhaps you'd finally found a good salad bar near your old job and now you have to start the search all over again. Or there weren't any bakeries near your previous office to tempt you and now there's one right on the corner. You'll have to establish new automatic behaviors to replace the ones that worked in the past.

Loss can also mess up your eating habits. If you lose a job and don't find another one soon enough, depression and self-doubt can make the refrigerator your favorite, friendly companion. You console yourself during all the extra hours at home by buying buckets of ice cream and bags of chips, not only that, but you might also lack the energy to be as active as you once were. Even worse, losing a family member or friend can completely devastate your life and diet. Once again, grief upends the order of daily activities, including what you eat. Many find comfort in what has not been lost: platters of food to fill the void.

Happily Fatter After

When it comes to Diet Busting life changes, marriage is in a category all its own. According to a study done by Jeffery Sobal, PhD, of Cornell University, "there is a definite relationship between marriage and weight gain." And another study done by Robert Jeffery, PhD, at the University of Minnesota School of Public Health in Minneapolis and reported in *Obesity Research* documented an average weight gain of six to eight pounds over a two-year period after getting married.

Marriage means more regular meals—especially meals in restaurants, which means more fatty foods and larger portions. But even when they're cooking at home, married people tend to prepare larger amounts of food, so portion size increases, and they pay less attention to what they're eating because they're dining with another person.

Additionally, people tend to take on the habits and patterns of their spouses. According to Sobal, one of the selection criteria used to pick your spouse is how he/she eats. "If you're a vegetarian, or a gourmet diner, you are more likely to feel comfortable with someone who shares your individual eating traits. Think about it—you're going to be eating with this person the rest of your life," says Sobal.

According to David L. Katz, MD, MPH, professor of public health at Yale University School of Medicine, one reason for weight gain after marriage is the "I've got him/her now, so I don't have to work so hard" mentality. He also suggests that "increased responsibilities, decreased leisure time, increased stress/financial pressure, and reduced time spent in athletic pursuits" are all factors. And finally, eating with another person "makes it okay" and more "fun" to consume "sin" foods like cookies, cakes, ice cream, and chips.

And what about becoming a parent? According to a study from Duke University Medical Center that appeared in the *Journal of Women's Health*, researchers found that women faced an average 7 percent increased risk of obesity per child born, and men an average of 4 percent.

"On top of the sleepless nights and irregular feeding schedules, there are real changes that couples undergo when starting a family that relate to their food and activity behavior. Couples spend more time at home and become less active, and this is the pattern that they tend to stick with," explains Lori Bastian, MD, MPH, associate professor of medicine at Duke University Medical Center. Additionally, fast food, nibbling here and there, and eating anything that's fast and tastes good become the norm. As for exercise, who has the time?

So, what can you do to avoid "The Wedding Waistline"?

Beware of Marital Sabotage: "One of the most common challenges to weight control in marriage is sabotage. This is when one of the pair is threatened by the weight-loss efforts of the other. The resultant behavior is an effort, subtle or not, to undermine the spouse, often by bringing 'seductive' foods into the home," says Katz. Also, many of our major activities involve food—romantic dinners, popcorn at the movies, socializing at restaurants—and "a partner can feel threatened that family fun will be thwarted. This builds a lot of resentment, making it a very emotional issue," says Cynthia Sass, MPH, MA, RD, author of *Your Diet Is Driving Me Crazy.*

Communicate: Let your partner know how important it is for you to lose weight.

Do It Together: Have your partner (and your entire family) eat healthier along with you. Studies have shown that partners who diet together lose more weight than those who don't. You can make it fun, taking low-fat cooking classes together, shopping for tasty low-calorie foods, and taking long, romantic walks.

Make It Separate: You don't always have to eat the same foods as your partner, meal after meal. Try to cook separately if your partner doesn't want to participate in healthier eating. For instance, you could both have chicken, one grilled and the other fried. When getting take-out, there is no rule that you have to order from the same place. And finally, when it comes to dining out, you could compromise, taking turns choosing the restaurant. This way, you have a chance to pick the healthier ones.

Prepare in Advance: If your spouse is a poor eater and won't exercise, be prepared. Think about your meals in advance; prepare for social occasions such as eating out or parties. Come up with strategies to help you stay in control—like keeping low-calorie fudge pops in the freezer for when your spouse is enjoying bowl after bowl of ice cream.

Avoid Parental Gain: Keep yourself conscious of not letting these "family additions" add to your waistline. Instead of fast food, use quick and easy low-calorie frozen dinners (e.g., Healthy Choice, Lean Cuisine, Smart Ones). Babies need fresh air, too—take long walks with your stroller. You might even want to invest in a jogging stroller. Keep in mind, if you're overweight, your kids will likely be overweight, too—they inherit more than just your genes. So be a positive role model of healthy eating for them.

Here are a few more classic Diet Buster moments, one or more of which might well ring a bell for you.

Special Occasions: Maybe you're always on a diet, but on special occasions like birthdays, family dinners, parties, or on dates, weddings, christenings, New Year's celebrations, birthdays, bar/bat mitzvahs, retirement dinners, you think it's okay to eat high calorie and high-fat foods. When I once added up my own roster of "special days" (including every event or inclination), the total came to about fifty days per year. The math tells the real story, though. If you ate just 500 extra calories on those days (which is not that hard—it's about one piece of cake or one bowl of ice cream), that would be about 25,000 calories, or more than seven pounds a year! Who would have thought that just letting go on a few special days could add up to so many pounds?

The truth is that *not* finding excuses to Diet Bust on special occasions can be the best celebration yet. The benefits will ultimately lead to a happier, more fulfilling, healthier life.

Weekends: Maybe you say, "I work hard at my job, live a busy life, and manage to diet all week long, but once the weekend rolls around, well, I like to live life. I'm not going to diet on the weekend." Sound familiar? The journal of *Obesity Research* looked at this phenomenon and reported that on the weekends (i.e., Friday through Sunday), we tend to eat an additional 115 calories per day, primarily from fat and alcohol, which is an extra 345 calories per week. This can add up to an additional five pounds in a year.

Watch Out for Weekends

According to Amy A. Gorin, PhD, an assistant professor of psychiatry and human behavior at Brown Medical School, one of the primary predictors of weight maintenance or gain is dietary consistency. Those who maintain the same diet regimen across the week and year are more likely to maintain their weight loss over the following year than those who dieted more strictly on weekdays and/or nonholiday periods. One possible explanation for this finding is that consistency in diet regimen is a characteristic that develops naturally over time in maintainers.

In the Workplace: Between workday pressures, social protocol, and those never-ending lunch meetings, it's no wonder the workplace can be a minefield of overeating opportunity! Whether it's bingeing on sweets, bagels, or baked goods that are lying around the office (especially to get through long mornings or the four o'clock slump), overeating at business meals or client functions, splurging at weekly lunches with your coworkers, stress eating throughout the day, grabbing unhealthy foods when you're on the go, or giving in to temptation at happy hour, many people experience their Diet Busters in the workplace.

Collective Eating: Do you like to eat, drink, and be merry? Believe it or not, these can be mutually exclusive events. Many people, however, experience their Diet Busters in the following ways: overeating when dining out; making poor choices off the menu; feeling social pressure when eating with certain groups of friends; engaging in unhealthy, if not mindless snacking at movies or sporting events; and eating breakfast, lunch, and dinner twice—once with your kids, then again with your spouse or friends.

Collective eating can even be as simple as eating with a friend or family member. We all have friends and family members who can eat whatever they want. It seems as if they don't absorb anything they put in their mouth, and eating with them can create a desire to partake in the food festivities. In fact, the research journal *Appetite* reported that whether a person ate in "the company of others, alone at work or in one's spare time turned out to be of decisive importance." The investigators found that when you eat with "familiar" people like family you tend to eat to excess.

Then there are the family and friends who are *food pushers*. These are the people who are always telling you that you look great, and in fact, "you're getting too thin." "How can one bite hurt?" they ask. Or, "It's a birthday party!" or "You have to at least have a taste."

In my family, we often joke that our minds are so involved with food that we're thinking about what to have for lunch before we've even finished breakfast.

Locations, Activities, and Times of Day: There are certain places that make me immediately think of food. My aunt's house is one of those places. The second I walk in the door, I somehow think I have a license to eat fattening foods—and she's got plenty of them ready to serve up. Everyone has food associations with certain places, activities, or even certain times of the day. Does a baseball game conjure up images of hot dogs and peanuts for you? Does a day at the beach *need* to be accompanied by ice cream with hot-fudge sauce? There are also situations like Scott's job-related travel. Whatever it is, for many of us there is a time, circumstance, situation, or event that inevitably causes us to bust our diet.

Now I'm going to ask you to identify your top Diet Buster moments; the circumstances, situations, or events that are—and probably always have been—most difficult for you. Doing that will reveal that these are *patterns of behavior*, not just isolated incidents, and that to lose and maintain your weight, you need to find ways to control them.

▸ During what situations, circumstances, or events do you continually find yourself slipping up on a weight-control plan?

▸ At what times do you feel you've lost control?

▸ At what point(s) do you typically feel guilty and disappointed about your choices?

▸ What can you do in the future to prepare yourself for these Diet Busting Moments?

Using the examples below as a guide, brainstorm *your* top Diet Buster Moments. For each one, write down three ways to prepare for the next time you are placed in that situation. Here's an example: *Whenever I go to my parents' home for a visit, I tend to eat candy, cakes, and ice cream. They have bowls filled with candies for my nieces and always have cake and ice cream for dessert. Each time I promise myself I won't, but then I eat all that sugar and fat anyway.*
In the Future:

i.   *When I go to my parents' house, I will bring healthy snacks and stock the refrigerator and pantry.*

ii. *I will also let my parents know that sticking to my Livable Diet is important to me and I would appreciate their not leaving bowls of candy out in front of me. I will see if they will help make adjustments when they can.*

iii. *I will bring my own low-calorie ice cream to eat while everyone is having dessert so that I can join them and still feel comfortable.*

Now write down *three* scenarios of your own in your notebook.
Diet Buster Moment
In the Future:

i.

ii.

iii.

If You Are Still Stuck,
Your Parents May Have the Answers

If you're still not sure you've properly identified your dieting patterns and traps, it might be a good idea to look to your parents for answers. The reality is that self-evaluation and reflection can be difficult.
That said, I'll let you in on a little trick-of-the-trade to ease the way: If
you want to hold up a mirror to examine your own, negative weight-
control and activity patterns and are having trouble seeing a clear reflection, turn the mirror just a bit so that it reflects your parents. As Carl
Jung pointed out, "Everything that irritates us about others can lead us
to an understanding of ourselves."

Between our genes and the way we were brought up (classic nature
plus nurture), it would seem obvious that our parents are the main
source of our current eating behaviors. Did they cause us to eat that extra slice of chocolate cake *today*, or to take the elevator instead of the
stairs? No, they didn't. Ultimately, as adults, we make our own choices.
Yet sometimes we realize, to our chagrin, that we're unconsciously following our parents' patterns. Like it or not, there are important lessons
to be learned from them.

As you grow up—especially if you spend your formative years with
your parents—you're not only developing your own unique positive
and negative patterns, you're also, consciously and unconsciously,
adopting many patterns from your parents. And, since it's easier to see
negative patterns in others than in yourself, examining *your parents' patterns* is a great place to start discovering your own.

Parents can have a have a significant influence on how we behave in
terms of diet and activity. As was reported in an article in the journal
Nurse Practitioner, ". . . the importance of familial and environmental influence is underscored with recognition that childhood is a critical period for shaping the dietary and lifestyle behaviors that can have
implications for adult, heart-disease risk." And in yet another article,
this one in *Pediatrics* magazine, researchers concluded that the eating
behaviors of children are influenced by parents and that, "parenting is
related to the other factors that influence eating behavior, including
modeling of eating behaviors" [emphasis added].

So, yes, your parents do influence your eating patterns, and looking
at *their* negative patterns offers another set of clues you can use to determine your own. Notice their behaviors and choices—what they order

at a restaurant, foods they have stocked in the kitchen, and how much they eat. It's a lot easier when you're studying someone else, isn't it?

But don't get me wrong. I'm not suggesting that your parents are responsible for your weight today. They are not to blame (you'll be learning more about blame in Step 7), but looking at them can help you to see the patterns you've been having trouble recognizing in yourself.

Take a look at the exercise below to see how your parents can help you to help yourself.

Do As I Say, Not As I Do

For this exercise, take out your notebook and write down *five* negative patterns of behavior related to eating, physical activity, and/or exercise that you see in your mother/father or the woman/man who most influenced you as you grew up (e.g., My mother/father always enjoyed a big slice of coffee cake after dinner or my mom/dad would refrain from eating desserts during the workweek, but when the weekend rolled around, like clockwork, he/she would binge and eat more than half a pie or a whole box of cookies, drink plenty of beer, go through bags of chips, and end Sunday with a huge dish of ice cream).

1 . . . 2 . . . 3 . . . 4 . . . 5 . . .

Now list the *five* negative eating, physical activity, and/or exercise patterns you see in them that you are most likely to duplicate or have duplicated. That is, basically, what eating/exercise behaviors have you copied from them?

1 . . . 2 . . . 3 . . . 4 . . . 5 . . .

Becoming Aware

While most of us do not expect perfection of ourselves in other aspects of our life, many of us feel we must carry out our weight-loss program to the letter. Perfection is unrealistic, but if you become aware of your Diet Busters and other Diet Traps, they won't have to be catastrophes or license to abandon your new lifestyle choice.

Too often, instead of getting back on the horse, so to speak, we use our lapses as opportunities to eat whatever we want. I can't even count the number of times when, after I had a slipup, I would continue eating "bad" foods—all the time telling myself "Hey, I've already blown it, why stop now."

Instead, give yourself a break and see your lapses for what they are: valuable opportunities to identify when and how you give in to temptation. The more you do that, the better able you'll be to keep a clear head when you feel one of those moments coming on and develop strategies for counteracting it and staying in control.

◀◀◀ STEP 6 ▶▶▶

Weave in Physical Activity

"What you have to do and the way you have to do it is incredibly simple. Whether you are willing to do it, that's another matter."
—Peter F. Drucker

Notice that this Step does not even *mention* the word *exercise* in the title. That's on purpose. Not because exercise isn't important, but because for my clients, and many other nonexercisers, it conjures up images of twenty-somethings with perfect bodies working out in a gym. So I use the term "physical activity" instead. Physical activity can refer to any kind of movement, whether it's organized or not. Duration is not important and neither is when or how it's accomplished.

I'm often amazed that clients who are ready, willing, and able to start doing things that might at first appear to be rather complicated, like reading labels and searching the supermarket shelves for Calorie Bargains or learning the nutritional values of various proteins, fats, and carbohydrates, seem totally flummoxed by how they can possibly increase their physical activity.

I'm here to tell you that it isn't difficult: There's no mystery involved. It's as simple as taking a walk.

You don't have to be an exercise junkie or a fanatic to reap the weight-loss benefits of physical activity. Burning off one hundred calories by walking for twenty-five minutes may not be as easy as cutting one hundred calories (one large bite of a candy bar) from your daily diet, but it is better, and healthier, to do both. In addition to which, increasing your physical activity will speed up your metabolism so that you use

Finding Your Resting Metabolic Rate (RMR)

Also known as the Resting Energy Expenditure, this is the rate at which you burn calories during a twenty-four-hour period in a nonactive state. Knowing your Resting Metabolic Rate is important because we burn about 75 percent of our calories in a nonactive state. There is research to indicate that increasing physical activity will slightly increase your RER/RMR. Not bad. As I've already shown, every little bit helps. The following is an equation (that can vary between 6 and 15 percent) that is frequently used to determine RER/RMR.

Harris-Benedict Equations (calories/day):

Step 1: Calculate your resting or basal metabolic rate (RMR)
Female: $655.1 + (4.35 \times$ weight in pounds$) + (4.699 \times$ height in inches$) - (4.676 \times$ age$)$
Male: $66.5 + (6.25 \times$ weight in pounds$) + (12.71 \times$ height in inches$) - (6.775 \times$ age$)$

Step 2: Calculate your caloric needs
Once you've arrived at this number, you can figure out how active you are and get an idea of how many calories in total you burn each day.

You can then determine your caloric needs by calculating your activity level.

Multiply your RER/RMR by the number given below for your level of activity.

Sedentary 1.2 (You sit, drive, lie down, or stand in one place for most of the day and don't do any type of exercise.)

Light Activity 1.3–1.4 (Sedentary for most of the day and do light activity, such as walking, for no more than two hours daily.)

Moderate Activity 1.5 (On your feet most of the work day, light lifting only, and no structured exercise.)

Very Active 1.6–1.7 (Typical workday includes several hours of physical labor, such as light industry and construction-type jobs.)

Extreme Activity 2–2.4 (Heavy manual labor; army and marine recruit training; competitive athlete.)

The result is the number of calories you burn each day. To lose weight, you will need to increase your level of activity and/or decrease your caloric intake until you are burning more calories than you consume.

more calories when you're *not* being physically active—which is when you burn about 75 percent of your caloric intake.

Every major study on weight control notes the value of making increased physical activity a part of your life, especially and specifically to prevent weight regain.

Rod Dishman, PhD, professor of exercise science at the University of Georgia reporting in the *Southern Medical Journal* showed that knowledge, attitudes, intentions, expected benefits, beliefs about personal control of health and fitness, perceived barriers to physical activity, and self-efficacy have all been associated with whether or not we increase our physical activity. The majority of the research, however, points to three major reasons why people *don't* increase their physical activity.

One is that we have both environmental and perceived personal barriers that cause us to believe it would be difficult and problematic to engage in regular physical activity. Our perceived personal barriers might include lack of time, health concerns, and lack of motivation. A report published in the *Journal of the American Association of Occupational Health Nurses* concludes that the primary reason for inactivity was lack of time. The most common environmental barriers, according to *Health Education Behavior* include safety, the lack of availability and/or cost of parks, beaches, recreation centers, pools, and fitness centers.

The *American Journal of Public Health*, reports that numerous studies have shown that people increase their physical activity (e.g., walk and cycle more) when their neighborhood is denser; that is, incorporating "a mixture of land uses (e.g., shops are within walking distance of homes) and connected streets (e.g., gridlike pattern instead of many cul-de-sacs). Other community design characteristics, such as the condition of sidewalks, the presence of bike paths, street design, traffic volume and speed, and crime, are hypothesized to be related to physical activity . . ."

Overcome Perceived Environmental Barriers to Physical Activity

Ask yourself the following questions about where you live:

1.   Does your neighborhood have public or private recreation facilities (such as public swimming pools, parks, walking trails, bike paths, activity centers, etc.)?

2. Are they in good condition? Can you see yourself using them?

3. Does your local public school have any facilities you can use?

4. Does your neighborhood shopping mall have any walking programs available?

5. Do you use nearby creeks, rivers, and lakes for water-related physical activities such as canoeing, kayaking, swimming, or water skiing (sorry, fishing doesn't cut it)?

6. Do concerns about safety at the public recreation facilities in your community influence your using them? Do you have safety concerns about walking in your neighborhood? Have you thought about how you can overcome these safety issues?

7. What are the names of the nearby parks? Walking/hiking trails? Bike paths?
   a.
   b.
   c.
   d.

To locate hiking and/or biking trails in your area, log on to wwww.traillink.com or www.pedbikeinfo.org.

8. Can you see yourself using any of the facilities mentioned above? If not, why?

9. What are you willing to do to increase your physical activity? What seems manageable and doable—something you can do automatically every day without fail?

Another important reason many people don't increase their physical activity is because they lack self-efficacy. The *American Journal of Health Promotion* reported that an increase in self-efficacy directly influences an increase in physical activity. What does self-efficacy mean? According to Albert Bandura, the Stanford University professor who coined the term, it refers to the *belief* in one's ability to "organize and execute" whatever it is one would like to do—meaning that if we want to accomplish increasing our physical activity, we first have to believe that we can do it.

Self-efficacy influences how we feel, the choices we make, the effort we exert, and the length of time we continue our physical activity. So how do you increase self-efficacy?

As you come to understand and accept the strategies, research information, and stories of client successes I'll be providing in this Step, you will gradually become persuaded and confident that you *can* weave physical activity into your life. And by that I don't mean working out on some fancy machine at a gym or performing in an aerobics class. I mean, quite literally, putting one foot in front of the other and doing something as simple as walking or increasing your steps during the regular course of your day. As you make attempts to do that, and as you become more proficient through these experiences, you will see that you *are* able to *get moving*. That's what increasing your self-efficacy is about. By understanding, reading, and becoming more aware that all you have to do is get out there, make a few adjustments in your life, and take a few more steps each day, you will see that increasing your level of physical activity is something you *can* do.

The last of the three major reasons we don't get moving is that we don't perceive the benefit of increasing physical activity. We really don't appreciate what it will do for us. No problem there, because by the time you finish this Step you will be thoroughly convinced of the benefit.

How do you increase your physical activity?

1. Find things you like to do—tennis, basketball, yoga, swimming, walking, racquetball, skiing—anything you can do on a regular basis.
2. Understand your environmental constraints and barriers. Learn how to work around them by setting goals and planning in advance (strategies you'll be learning more about in Step 8). Research your area. Find walking and hiking trails, figure out what you're going to do on a regular basis. Also, keep in mind that it doesn't have to be the same thing every day. You can have a walk one day, and on the other days simply go window-shopping or increase your activity in some of the other ways we'll be discussing in this Step.
3. Remember that small increases in activity, such as taking the stairs instead of the elevator or parking at the farthest distance from the store in the mall, make a big difference.

4. Use the Excuse Busters you'll be getting in Step 7 to overcome your excuses. Since the number one excuse for not exercising or increasing physical activity is lack of time, look for opportunities to make time for weaving physical activity into your life.

5. Motivation is important when it comes to physical activity, so think about what will keep you going. Make sure that you pick an activity that's exciting and rewarding *to you*.

6. Don't leave your increase in physical activity up to chance; make it easy. Create automatic-exercise opportunities. Use exercise videos, walking clubs, hiking, and home-fitness equipment. Read Step 8 on the Power of Planning. Physical activity needs to be just like brushing your teeth. Figure out ways to do it every day.

7. Use the information in Step 9 to mentally rehearse how you will increase your physical activity—think of every last detail, such as putting on your sneakers, picking up your tennis racket, getting out the bike. Plan exactly how you will fit these activities into your life. These techniques will help to get you going and create the automatic behavior that you're looking for.

The Benefits of Physical Activity

Study after study shows that increasing physical activity has tremendous health advantages. Just take a look at all these benefits:

▸ Helps develop lean muscle and reduce body fat

▸ Increases the number of calories you burn while you're doing nothing (RMR)

▸ Reduces the risk of dying from coronary heart disease and developing high-blood pressure, colon cancer, and diabetes

▸ Increases energy and flexibility

▸ Helps maintain healthy bones, muscles, and joints

▸ Reduces symptoms of tension, anxiety, and depression, and fosters improvement in mood and feelings of well-being, self-esteem, and improved body image

▸ Increases mental alertness

These are all great benefits, but one of the most important reasons to increase your physical activity is that it will help you lose weight and, more important, *it will prevent you from regaining any weight you have actually lost.*

I tell you this based on my own experience, feedback from clients, and the research that has appeared in most of the significant scientific journals. In fact, in a review of several major studies on long-term weight maintenance, James W. Anderson reported in the *American Journal of Clinical Nutrition* that those who substantially increased their physical activity were clearly more successful in maintaining their weight loss than were the groups with lower levels of physical activity.

It's a simple mathematical formula. If there are 3,500 calories to a pound of fat, burning just an additional one hundred calories per day means losing about ten pounds in one year. Dr. James Hill, founder of the National Weight Loss Registry, has found that those who successfully sustained significant weight loss—keeping off more than sixty pounds for at least five years—had increased their daily physical activity by approximately sixty minutes each day. And according to John M. Jakicic, PhD, a professor at the University of Pittsburg reporting in *Endocrinology and Metabolism Clinics of North America,* exercise should be progressively increased to approximately 300 minutes per week (60 min × 5 d/wk) to optimize the impact of exercise on body-weight regulation. But again, that doesn't mean you have to be sweating in a gym. The Pound of Prevention study conducted by the School of Public Health at the University of Minnesota has shown that any increased physical activity, whether moderate (i.e., walking and home-maintenance activities such as gardening or snow shoveling), high intensity (i.e., running/jogging, biking, swimming, exercise classes), or tied to occupation (e.g., construction worker versus office worker) was a predictor of future weight loss and weight maintenance.

In a key study published in the *Journal of the American Medical Association,* Ross E. Andersen, PhD, a professor at Johns Hopkins University School of Medicine also showed that a program of diet plus lifestyle activity may offer similar health benefits and be a suitable alternative to diet plus vigorous activity for overweight individuals. The diet-plus-lifestyle program was as effective as the diet-plus-aerobic training program in improving weight, systolic blood pressure, and serum lipid and lipoprotein levels among these individuals. Participants in their team were advised to increase their levels of moderate-intensity physical activity by thirty minutes per day on most days of the week. They were taught to incorporate short bouts of activity into their daily schedules, for example, walking instead of driving short distances and taking stairs instead of the elevator.

Find Your Activity Opportunities

To discover where your own opportunities lie, you first need to evaluate what you typically do in a day (which means *all your activities* right down to how you shop and clean) and then look for ways to incorporate increased physical activity into your life.

Take Brenda, for instance, a client from the outskirts of Sarasota, Florida. Brenda wasn't really sure exactly how to do this. We needed to *write* down what an average week looked like for her. A typical suburbanite, she drove everywhere she could. If she had to go to the post office, even though it was down the street, she would drive. To her, walking was out of the question. There were time issues, and she felt self-conscious walking in her neighborhood because no one else did *and* because she was overweight. But the one thing she was willing to do was to start using a bicycle for many of her local errands. Her local streets were very bike friendly because there were two schools in the neighborhood, and she even thought biking might actually be more convenient than driving in some instances. She purchased an inexpensive bike with saddlebag-type baskets on the back, and after a while she found herself using the bicycle all the time. She lost thirty pounds and, since she's continued to bike, she's maintained the loss. Now she's even started to walk on a regular basis.

Here are a few quick-and-easy examples of ways to increase physical fitness through daily activities. Use these suggestions to inspire you to investigate and determine your own physical activity opportunities; *that's the way to make it automatic.*

Mow it: Save money and mow your own lawn. And that doesn't mean using a lawn tractor or a mower you ride on, it means using the motorized push-type mower. In half an hour, you could burn about 175 calories.

Use the pet: Studies have shown that almost 60 percent of dog owners do not walk their pets. Instead, they let them out in the backyard on their own. Take the time to go for a long walk with your dog each and every day. A thirty-minute stroll with your pooch burns up to eighty calories.

Wash your car: Here's another opportunity to save money and burn calories at the same time. Half an hour with soap sponge or chamois burns about 140 calories. Keep a very clean car and you could lose seven to ten pounds a year!

Leave the car at home: A couple of days a week, if the weather permits, leave your car at home and either walk, bike, or take mass transportation to work.

Dish it out: Washing the dishes and cleaning the house for an hour will burn more than one hundred calories, which may make such tasks seem more worth while.

Gardening: Get out the shovel and start a garden. And while you're at it, try growing some healthy food! Thirty minutes of gardening burns about 160 calories.

Other Ways to Increase Your Activity

▸ Walk to the farthest restroom at work
▸ Have meetings while going for a walk
▸ Play with your children and/or grandchildren
▸ Go to the mall with the intention of walking and window shopping for sixty minutes three times a week. Leave your wallet home.
▸ Don't use the drive-thru windows at banks or fast-food restaurants. Park and walk inside.

---

*If you're already doing these things, that's wonderful, but remember, they don't count as an increase in physical activity. You have to **add new activities** to increase your caloric expenditure.*

This may seem obvious, but it's an important concept considering that the scientific journal *Health Education Behavior* has found that while some people might not identify themselves as "exercisers," they claim to get enough physical activity just from "caregiving, housekeeping, and workday activities." The problem is that they need to *increase* these activities if they are to have an effect on their weight.

Calorie Burning per Minute of Exercise			
	Easy	*Moderate*	*Brisk/Fast*
Walking	4 cal/min	4.5 cal/min	5 cal/min
Biking	7 cal/min	11cal/min	13.5 cal/min
Running	9 cal/min	13 cal/min	15 cal/min

Not convinced yet? Then you might want to consider another study undertaken at the University of Pittsburgh, which found that easy physical activity burns calories and aids weight loss just as effectively as high-intensity exercise. Researchers followed 201 women ages 21 to 45 throughout a year. Two groups were formed—one walked off 1,000 calories per week and the other walked off 2,000 calories per week. Those in the 1,000-calorie variable shed an average of 13 pounds; the 2,000-calorie group lost about twenty pounds—the weight was lost regardless of the participants' pace during their walks. This means that slow walkers can burn calories despite their slower pace. It will just take them longer than brisk walkers to lose the weight.

Given this information, it's not surprising that a study published in the *American Journal of Public Health* and *American Journal of Health Promotion* found that people who live in the suburbs—and therefore drive everywhere—weigh 6.3 pounds more than urbanites, who are able to walk more in dense cities. So what should you do? How about taking a walk! According to the National Weight Control Registry, 77 percent of successful weight losers use walking as their primary means of physical activity.

Amazing Ultra-Fabulous Walking!

It's very hard for me to convince people that doing something as simple as taking a walk can really contribute not only to their health but also to their weight loss. And, I must say, I never thought much of walking myself—I mean, it was always a necessary means to an end if I had to get from point A to point B. But, I must admit it's truly an amazing activity—yes, *walking* is an activity. Walking is an art in itself. My morning strolls have now become a time to relax and meditate. There is nothing like going for a nice walk. You can do it anywhere. And you can accomplish other tasks at the same time, such as picking up your cleaning, shopping, or picking up a quart of milk. Walking is one of the most important life-changing physical activities I've been able to offer my clients.

And, get this, you burn only about 20 percent more calories when you run a mile than you do when you walk a mile. Less sweat as well as less muscle and joint stress at about the same calorie expenditure. Not bad, right?

In fact, recent studies have shown the many benefits of walks. Walking has fewer risks than fast-paced jogging; walkers get a better and fuller overall workout than most runners; and age does not serve as an impediment—both young and old can participate and reap the rewards.

Connie, a client of mine, was truly averse to increasing her physical activity—for her it was "just too hard to find the time" and when she'd tried to start a walking program in the past, it never seemed to work out. She would get all excited in the beginning, but after a few weeks, the second she started to become busy, the walk was the first thing out the window. Our goal was to try and figure out how to incorporate walking into her everyday life—combining organized walking or hiking with functional walking, such as a trip to the grocery store. First of all, it was important for Connie to understand that just because it hadn't worked before didn't mean it wasn't going to work this time. When we looked into her past failures, it became clear that, although time was a factor, the more important reason she was unsuccessful was that she'd never really preplanned her walking routes and hadn't incorporated socialization into her walks—that is, walking with another person who would help to motivate her. So Connie came up with five different, safe, scenic, and accessible routes she could use. Some were in her neighborhood, so she could use them when she was in a time crunch; others she would have to drive to, but they were in places she had to be anyway (picking up her children, shopping, going to the video store, etc.). At first, she convinced two of her neighbors to accompany her on her local walks, and after a while, they occasionally began to accompany her to the off-site routes as well.

She also started using a pedometer and a calendar, on which she kept track of how many steps she took on the days she didn't follow one of her predetermined routes. She stopped marking the calendar after the first six months, but she's been able to sustain her walking program and is still going strong. She loves it and no longer feels pushed for time—in fact, she doesn't think about it all, she just does it.

Let's face it, the majority of Americans cannot run for thirty minutes straight. Health programs understand the couch-potato epidemic and are now launching several, well-publicized step-awareness programs like America on the Move, which aspires to get people to add two thousand additional steps—that's about one mile—to their daily routine. Another, much bolder step program, Shape Up America!, strives to get Americans to walk ten thousand steps a day, or about five miles. Malls, parks, and even your very own neighborhood's sidewalks are perfect sites for a ten-, fifteen-, or even thirty-minute walk. On rainy days, malls can be converted into indoor tracks. Walk the entire mall for a good thirty minutes at a moderate speed. The level flooring (fewer injuries) and air conditioning are excellent motivators for using the mall as a walking spot. And you'll also have the benefit of people watching (which will make the time fly by) as well as fantasizing about all the great clothes you'll be able to buy—in a smaller size—when you've reached your weight-loss goal. Or, if walking around the mall isn't your thing, try locating walking tours around your city. Sightseeing is very distracting and before you know it, you'll have walked a few miles while discovering more about your neighborhood or even new neighborhoods.

Scenic routes are wonderful for hikes. Some parks even offer trails specifically designed for hikers. Grass and dirt paths are flat and reduce shock and stress on your feet. If you want to increase the difficulty factor, find paths with hills, take a few breaks, and walk for an hour instead of just thirty minutes. Or just increase the speed at which you walk.

Certain communities have walking clubs; take advantage of those resources and join. Walking in a group will increase motivation and distraction, and will help you to challenge yourself by keeping up with the others. Walk your dog, explore your parks, anything that will increase the number of steps you take throughout your day.

But before you go outside and start counting your steps, keep in mind that your choice of shoes is quite important. Podiatrists suggest getting cross trainers, running shoes, or walking shoes; however, stay away from those aesthetic shoes that are "all looks but no support."

Self-Monitoring

Want to improve your chances of sticking to your newly "woven-in" physical activity? Studies have shown that people who use some kind of self-monitoring device tend to stay with a program of physical activity longer than those who don't, because they have a way to measure their progress, which gives them a sense of accomplishment. "You could simply take a calendar and mark the days you exercise with a big X," says Carl Foster, PhD, professor of exercise science at the University of Wisconsin-LaCrosse. Or you could use a pedometer, as Connie did. Other ways of self-monitoring include keeping a diary or using a heart-rate monitor, an accelerometer (calorie tracker), or the calorie and mileage displays on cardiovascular equipment. So keep track of what you do, it helps keep you motivated.

Use a Pedometer to Self-Monitor

With the step craze sweeping America, new and more sophisticated tools have been developed and tailored for the growing population of walkers. The importance of self-monitoring lies in the fact that you will become aware of what your body is capable of doing, and once you are in tune with your body's capabilities, you can then increase your threshold, in this case by increasing the number of steps you take in a day.

Pedometers gained popularity with the advent of the 10,000 Steps goal for daily walking, an idea born forty years ago in Japan. The Japanese named their pedometers *manpo-kei*, meaning literally "10,000 steps meter." The idea was to make it easy for individuals to increase their activity without thinking too much. All they needed was a simple pedometer.

What Is a Pedometer?

A pedometer's basic function is to count steps. Pedometers contain an internal lever that is triggered by your hip movement, counting each one as a step. Most of the time, your pedometer will be counting your actual steps, but other movements can also cause the lever to go up and down—such as pulling up your pants, bending over to tie your shoe, even going over a pothole when you're riding in a car.

How Many Steps?

So how many steps are enough? "The average person accumulates three thousand to five thousand steps per day," says David R. Bassett, Jr., PhD, professor of health and exercise science at the University of Tennessee, Knoxville. The goal is to increase your number of steps per day to about ten thousand.

My advice—take it slowly, first doing a test with the pedometer for a week to evaluate your current number of steps. Then try to increase your steps by about 20 percent per month—all the while ensuring your newfound changes are sustainable. As a point of reference, depending on walking speed, you might walk between 96 and 120 steps each minute. You can easily see how these steps can add up.

Accuracy

"Pedometers can be off by as much as 40 percent," says Bassett. In fact, in his most recent study, which was published in *Medicine and Science in Sports and Exercise*, he rated the top pedometers for accuracy and reliability. In another study, Catrine Tudor-Locke, PhD, FACSM, professor of health promotion at Arizona State University, found a difference of 1,800 steps, or about one mile, between two pedometers over the course of a day.

What makes the difference? According to Dr. Bassett, Japan is one of the only countries that manufactures accurate pedometers. They actually have industry standards for pedometer production, and they are typically accurate to within 3 percent.

Unfortunately, there are only a few models available in the US that meet these standards, and they are imported from Japan. One such model, the Digi-Walker SW-200, is distributed by a company called New Lifestyles and costs about $22 (www.digiwalker.com). Accusplit (www.accusplit.com) sells the Japanese-made AE120, as well as other models made in Taiwan and China, which can be off by as much as 15 percent. The pedometer made for the national, public-health program America on the Move (the AX120) is produced in China and isn't nearly as accurate as the Japanese ones.

I did an informal "walk test" with a few of these devices by walking for 2.75 miles. Here are the results:

—GPS Garmin Frontrunner: 2.75 miles
—McDonald's Step With It pedometer: 3.0 miles
—Digi-Walker SW-200: 2.75 miles
—Accusplit (AX120): 2.6 miles

Now, if you own a pedometer that is not 100 percent accurate (many are not), don't despair. It doesn't mean you have to throw yours out and buy a new one. It simply means you need to realize that your pedometer may be overestimating or underestimating your actual steps, and to account for that, you may need to take more or fewer steps to reach the recommended ten thousand.

Other Tips

Wear it correctly. Pedometers need to be placed on your belt and should always be vertical. They will not be accurate if they are hanging over the side of your belt or waistline. Bassett recommends getting as close as possible to the midline of your body so that your pedometer can accurately record the steps from both feet. But again, make sure that your belly doesn't tip it over. Additionally, if you wear it on your pocket, its accuracy will be compromised.

Test it. "You shouldn't need to calibrate your pedometer. It should be good to go right out of the box," says Bassett. But always test your pedometer by putting it on, making sure it's comfortable, and going for a twenty-step walk test. If the reading is off by more than one step (5 percent error) and you're concerned about accuracy, repeat the test. If it's still off, you might want to return it for another. Your pedometer should work on any terrain, and it doesn't matter what type of shoe you're wearing. "Also, your pedometer should have a way of protecting its reset button during the day—if you get bumped and you lose all your data, that can be pretty disappointing," says Tudor-Locke.

What About Other Devices?

With a cost of about $25 to $30, pedometers are one of the least expensive tools for measuring distance. There are other more sophisticated devices, but they're more expensive. If you want more, try Nike's SDM Tailwind. Bassett recommends this type of unit, especially if you're going to use it for walking and running. "It's more accurate because it measures the forward and backward movement of the shoe," he explains. You strap it to your shoelace and it gives your total time, average pace, exact distance, and calories burned. It retails for about $115.

Another model I tested is the Garmin Forerunner 201, which was quite impressive if you can get over its limitations. It offers athletes an easy-to-read display, an ergonomic wristband, and an integrated global positioning system (GPS) sensor that provides precise speed, distance, and pace data. It's compact, easy to use, lightweight, and very accurate. I must say that I used it for about a month and enjoyed every minute of it. The problem is that there are times that the GPS signal is unavailable, and it only works outdoors. It retails for about $160.

Summary of 2004 Study's Top Pedometers

The most recent study conducted at the University of Tennessee found that the Lifecorder, the Digi-Walker SW-200, the New-Lifestyles NL-2000, and the Digiwalker SW-701 were the most accurate and reliable of thirteen brands. The Sportline 330 also made the top five, but did not meet the researchers' standards due to poor performance in another study.

Top 4 Accuracy and Reliability Combined

1. Kenz Lifecorder ($200)
2. Digi-Walker SW-200 ($22)
3. New-Lifestyles NL-2000 ($54)
4. Digi-Walker SW-701 ($30)

Overestimated Steps

1. Walk4Life LS 2525
2. Omron HJ-105
3. Oregon Scientific PE316CA

Underestimated Steps

1. Freestyle Pacer Pro
2. Accusplit Alliance 1510
3. Yamax Skeletone EM-180
4. Colorado on the Move
5. Sportline 345

Schneider PL, Crouter SE, Bassett DR. "Pedometer measures of free-living physical activity: comparison of thirteen models." *Medicine and Science in Sports and Exercise* 36 (2):331–35. Used with permission.

Do You Need a Heart-Rate Monitor?

The primary purpose of a heart-rate monitor is to gain a better understanding of your exercise intensity. "This is specifically important if you are a high-performance, competitive athlete. Knowing your heart rate and exercise intensity can determine where your anaerobic threshold exists (when your muscles start to get tired). From that point, with proper training, you can increase that threshold, and sustain peak performance for longer periods," says Walter Thompson, PhD, professor of exercise science at Georgia State University.

And what if you're just an occasional exerciser or just starting an exercise program? "Many times, beginner participants may not be aware of what it means to exercise at a moderate intensity, which in turn will affect their workout," says Carla B. Sottovia, PhD, the fitness director at the Cooper Fitness Center, Dallas, Texas.

In fact, if you exercise too hard, you will most likely quit before you get real benefits (and it could be dangerous). But if you know when to stop pushing, you can exercise for longer periods of time, get in better shape, and achieve greater exercise benefits.

A heart-rate monitor can help you determine if you are exercising too much, but you can also do the talk test. "Try reciting something you know really well while exercising, such as the Pledge of Allegiance. *If you can speak comfortably without any problems, you're doing just fine* and are probably in the 50 to 80 percent range. If you waffle a bit, you are probably working at 80 to 90 percent of your maximum heart rate. If you can't talk at all, you're above 90," says Foster.

If You Don't Work Out for at Least Sixty Minutes, Why Bother?

Not true, although I'm sure plenty of us would love to think that if we can't do sixty minutes of intense training a day, it's not worth doing any exercise. Why the confusion? Well, it's understandable given the mixed messages that are out there. The National Academy of Sciences' Institute of Medicine (IOM) recommends an hour each day of moderately intense physical activity to maintain cardiovascular health at a maximal level (and for maximum weight loss and weight control). But, on the other hand, the American College of Sports Medicine and the United States Surgeon General both recommend approximately thirty minutes of exercise three to five days a week for decreased disease risk and increased longevity.

"The reality is, for the average person who's getting little to no daily exercise, anything is better than nothing. You can even benefit from doing ten minutes of daily walking or some other low intensity exercise," says Walter R. Thompson.

Continuous Physical Activity Is Not Necessary

And what if you exercised for ten minutes three times a day instead of thirty minutes all at once—is that really just as effective?

Yes, according to a number of studies, including one published in *Medicine and Science in Sports and Exercise* that looked at one group of twenty-four sedentary women who walked thirty minutes all at once five days a week, and a second group who walked three times a day for ten minutes (also five days a week). The improvements in cardiovascular fitness were virtually identical in the two groups.

"You can do aerobic training all at once or break it up into smaller chunks throughout the day. The health and fitness benefits are about the same," explains Steve Farrell, PhD, of the Cooper Institute in Dallas, Texas.

The problem is that, from a practical perspective, if you break up your physical activity, you might have a tendency to say, "Well, I was moving all day, so I'm getting all the exercise I need." You have to be aware of who you are and what works best for you. Some people do fine increasing their activity in small doses, fitting in ten minutes here and there. Others need to get it out of the way all at once.

In-Home Fitness Equipment

John M. Jakicic, PhD, in a study reported in the *Journal of the American Medical Association,* found that having home fitness equipment of any kind makes exercise more convenient and facilitates an increase in physical activity. That doesn't mean you have to go out and buy an expensive treadmill; you can simply get a few dumbbells and a few fitness videos, but if you do decide to buy, here's some advice.

Consumer Reports recently reviewed some of the top sellers, and unfortunately, the best ones are a bit expensive. For aerobics, the Treadclimber by Nautilus (TC3000) tested very well and costs $2,000 (800-436-7114). For strength training, *Consumer Reports* recommends the Bowflex Power Pro XTLU, also expensive at $1,750 (888-577-1052). For a bit less money, you can go with the Crossbow by Weider (WESY5983) for $695 (800-260-8996). As for abdominal devices and bun and thigh machines, don't bother—*Consumer Reports* couldn't recommend any of them.

Does this mean you have to spend a fortune on fitness equipment for the home? Not really. You can get a bicycle. Giant makes a great beach bike called the Simple Cruiser for around $200. It's comfortable, lightweight, and made for anyone, not just athletes. You can buy a wind trainer, which is a kind of stand you can attach to your bike to turn it into a stationary bicycle to use in inclement weather (e.g., CycleOps **Wind Trainer** $129.95). You can also get other workout classics like cast-iron dumbbells, which cost about $.50 per pound (i.e., a pair of twenty-pound weights would cost $20). Neoprene dumbbells are a little pricier at $1 per pound. For women, three-, five-, and eight-pound weights are typically appropriate, and ten-, fifteen-, twenty-five-, and thirty-pound weights for men.

Exercise balls are also inexpensive at about $20 to $35, but remember to buy the optional pump for an additional $15 (www.fitball.com). Another hot product that is regaining popularity is the medicine ball—yes, a medicine ball—which runs anywhere from $15 to $50 (www.thesportsauthority.com). But make sure you buy the workout books that go with them. Those will cost an additional $8 to $10.

Find out if you have the space for a home gym at www.precor.com—go to the Space Planner section, under Fitness Tools, it's really easy and fun to use.

And What About Sweating—Do I Have to Sweat?

I have a friend who believes that if he isn't sweating, he's not getting the exercise he needs and not losing weight. Unfortunately, sweating doesn't mean that you're burning calories. "Sweating is the way your body cools itself. Post-exercise weight loss often represents a loss of fluids from the body, not a reduction of fat," says Dr. Thompson. "People sweat because their body temperature increases—often times when you work out, your body temperature goes up and that's why sweating is associated with exercise. But that's where the relationship ends."

Actually, if you are just beginning an exercise program and you're sweating excessively, you should be very concerned. "It's a real mistake to monitor your level of exercise by how much you're sweating because excessive sweating can bring on heat exhaustion, followed by heat stroke," cautions Dr. Thompson. Experts suggest focusing on replacement of fluids rather than on the alleged pounds lost. For every pound you lose following exercise, you should drink at least twenty-four ounces of fluid.

Exercise Truths and Myths

Exercising Makes You Eat Right

I only wish that were true. Wouldn't it be nice if you started exercising and some hormone was released that forced you to eat better? Sure, it makes sense that if you start working out, you might want to take better care of yourself and eat less. But that isn't always the case. "The general public believes that they will improve their eating habits automatically when exercising, but this spontaneous healthy change just doesn't happen," says Joseph E. Donnelly, exercise physiologist at the University of Kansas in Lawrence. In fact, the reverse could actually occur. "People tend to think, 'I'm exercising and burning more calories, so I can eat whatever I want,'" says Donnelly. "Exercise is great, but it is not a panacea."

One reason this myth has been perpetuated could be due to workout fanatics. These people typically pay more attention to their eating habits and overall lifestyle choices. "But for the average person just starting out, this doesn't happen—you need to consciously work on changing both eating and activity habits," adds Donnelly.

To Burn the Most Calories, Don't Eat Before You Exercise

False. You don't burn more calories by *not* eating before you go out for your morning jog. In fact, the opposite is true. "If you don't eat, you won't have the energy to exercise as long, so you will burn fewer calories, not more," says Nancy Clark, MS, RD, author of *The Sports Nutrition Guidebook*. Clark recommends eating about 200 to 300 calories within the hour before exercising. So if you are exercising at four in the afternoon, you should have your calories between three and four PM. What if you exercise first thing in the morning? "Even eating a piece of fruit five minutes before you exercise, to get your blood sugar back up to normal, would be helpful. You need energy to get yourself moving and to make your workout more enjoyable and sustainable," says Clark.

What should you eat? "Try to have high-density carbohydrates, like an apple, some whole-grain cereal, or a banana," says Clark. Keep in mind, these calories shouldn't be in addition to your normal diet, just redistributed from your other meals or snacks.

**If You Are Not in the Fat-Burning Zone,
You Are Not Going to Lose Weight**

False. When heart-rate monitors became popular, the concept of the "fat-burning zone" emerged—claiming that if you worked out at a low-to-moderate intensity, your body would burn more fat than if you exercised at a higher intensity. To this day, most cardiovascular fitness equipment charts your fat-burning heart-rate zone for you. As pleasant as this idea might be, it's a complete myth.

Yes, you do burn a higher percentage of calories from fat when your body is at a lower heart rate. "The problem is, that's only half the equation. You may be burning more fat on a percentage basis, but you will be burning fewer calories overall, and the key to weight loss is caloric expenditure, *not fat burning*." says James Churilla, MS, RCEP, an exercise physiologist at Broward General Medical Center. "Given the same duration, working out at a higher intensity burns more calories (and fat), even though the percentage of fat burned may be lower." Here's an example to help illustrate this point: thirty minutes of walking burns about 200 calories (70 percent from fat or about 140 fat calories), whereas thirty minutes of jogging burns 300 calories (50 percent from fat or about 150 fat calories). So, you see, the higher-intensity jogging burns more calories *and* fat.

Muscle Turns to Fat Without Exercise

False again. Muscle is muscle and fat is fat. You can't transform one into the other. "Muscle atrophies—that is, gets smaller—and fat accumulates, usually as a result of less activity and the same amount of eating, which might give the appearance that muscle turns to fat," says John Acquaviva, PhD, professor of health and human performance at Roanoke College.

Motivation to Exercise

Once you've started to increase your physical activity and see the benefits from doing that, you may still need motivation to continue, or you may be inclined to actually start an organized exercise *program*. My clients often ask me what they can do to stay motivated once they've made the decision to get started.

Most experts say the key is to make exercise intrinsic—or internally motivated. "To really keep an exercise program going, it needs to be something you're doing because you value the actual activity—you appreciate the exercise for the sake of exercising," says Richard M. Ryan, PhD, a professor of psychology at the University of Rochester.

The bottom line: Physical activity doesn't have to be a horrible experience, and with more than 50 percent of people dropping out of their newfound exercise programs after only a few months, it's time to come up with a new routine.

Enjoy It: Focus on the enjoyment, feelings of competence, and social interaction that come from the experience. A study in the *International Journal of Sports Psychology* showed that a group who participated in aerobic exercise to improve their physical appearance didn't stick with it nearly as long as a group who did martial arts because they enjoyed it. And if you can't find something that you love right away, at the very least find something you don't hate. It's important to find as many redeeming qualities as possible for any of the exercises that you choose. And a study in *Health Education Research* also reported that the activity you decide to increase should be chosen carefully, with an emphasis on moderation in intensity and integration into your lifestyle—don't just start to increase your physical activity doing something you don't like.

Experiment and Match: Try a variety of activities. If you don't like to walk, how about biking, dancing, hiking, or golf? To spice things up, try listening to music or watching TV while you're working out. Most of us have tried exercises and probably became fatigued, disgusted, and just didn't like them—you need to set the bar a bit lower. There is an exercise for everyone, you just have to find the one that you love.

Avoid Rewards: I know it sounds strange, but researchers at the University of Rochester have compiled some very convincing evidence to indicate that you should not give yourself rewards for exercising. "Giving yourself or receiving rewards takes your eye off the ball—it gives you the wrong focus. Believe me, most rewards are not potent enough to get you on the treadmill at six o'clock every single morning for the rest of your life," says Dr. Ryan. If you really need rewards to get you moving, try to use them only in the beginning stages—until it becomes a habit. Remember that if you reach your goal, don't use rewards that go against your goal (e.g., an ice-cream sundae)—perhaps a massage would be a better choice.

Go Slow: People who tell me they want to start exercising often have grandiose ideas of getting up every morning, going to the gym, and then running five miles. Start off slowly if you've never been physically active before—even two or three times a week is better than nothing. In the initial stages, you really need to cut yourself a bit of slack, meaning if you miss a day or so, don't give up completely.

Excuses, Excuses, Excuses: We have many great excuses why we *can't* increase our physical activity, ranging from time constraints, lack of money, lack of energy, no place to do it, bad weather, and physical discomfort. Do you have excuses? Go right to Step 7 and learn how to bust your excuses. But just to give you a preview: Brainstorm and write down all the reasons you can think of for *not* working toward your fitness goals. Remember to include your self-doubts, fears, and insecurities—these are excuses too! Be honest. Next, punch holes in your excuses until they are no longer airtight. Do this by coming up with counterarguments for every single excuse you may have for not exercising—this is called Excuse Busting (coming up in the next Step).

Make It Social: There is a plethora of research demonstrating that working out with a group on a regular basis increases your likelihood of sticking with your routine. One study found that married couples who worked out together had a significantly higher attendance and lower dropout rate than married people who worked out alone. Find a regular fitness class that you know you'll enjoy. Organize a group of friends, coworkers, or neighbors to participate in some regular fitness activity. Get yourself a workout buddy. Not only will you increase your fitness level and improve your appearance, but you'll also reduce stress and increase the effectiveness of your immune system (social groups do that)—and you will probably have a good time as well.

Have a Plan and Set Goals: Don't just decide that "starting next week" you're going to walk every day—especially if you don't like walking. Investigate your options, write them down, and make the decision as if it's something that's important to you. Come up with a plan for exercise that will keep you excited for longer than twenty-four hours. Powerful Planning in Step 8 will help you with this planning and goal setting. Keep in mind that one of the most important things is to remain flexible with everything—including your exercise, your time, and yourself.

Visualize Your Future: Being able to see yourself in a positive situation in the future will keep you focused on your exercise path. Create a Life Preserver—that is, an imagined future event in which you have achieved your fitness goal. For example, think of the excitement you will have after completing your first two-hour hike or finishing a scenic, bike tour. Learn more about creating a Life Pre-server, using visualization and mental rehearsal to increase exercise adherence in Step 9, Think—and Make It Happen.

Subtle Reminders

Magazines and newsletters are terrific reminders and motivators—they're inexpensive, and with a new issue every month, they're truly the gift that keeps on giving. Plus, magazines and newsletters are always running specials and free offers, so maybe you can get a free subscription for a friend and get him or her motivated, too. In terms of selecting magazines that are inspiring, motivating, and packed with high-quality information, my picks for women are *Prevention, Fitness, Self,* and *Shape,* and specifically for men, *Men's Health* and *Men's Fitness* are the best out there, hands down.

As for newsletters, *Food & Fitness Advisor* by Weill Medical College of Cornell University offers cutting-edge nutrition and health information (annual subscription $39.00; available by calling 800-829-2505 or on the Internet at http://foodandfitnessadvisor.com/), while the *Tufts University Health & Nutrition Letter* (annual subscription $28.00; http://www.healthletter.tufts.edu/) and the *Nutrition Action Healthletter* from the Center for Science in the Public Interest (circ@cspinet.org) have excellent advice in an easy-to-read format.

Get Fancy—Try Strength Training

I'm not suggesting that everyone *has to* embark on a program of strength training in order to lose weight. I said at the beginning of this Step that it was going to be about increasing your level of physical activity in a way that worked for you—and I meant that. But it's also true that the more you are able to do, the greater the rewards you'll enjoy in terms of both weight loss and overall health. So, for those of you who think you might want to do something more, I'm including strength training as an option to consider. The purpose of lifting weights is not so you can eventually move a refrigerator, but to reap the substantial health benefits, which include:

▶ Strengthening bones, muscles, and connective tissue, which decreases your risk of injury (and osteoporosis)

▶ Preventing the loss of muscle mass. Adults lose about a pound of muscle mass per year, and muscle tissue is partly responsible for the number of calories burned at rest (the resting metabolic rate, or RMR)

By increasing your muscle mass, you increase your RMR, and make it easier to maintain a healthy body weight. In fact, for every one pound of muscle tissue you gain through strength training you will burn an additional thirty to fifty calories per day. Think of that—fifty calories per day is equal to 18,250 calories per year or about 5.2 pounds.

▶ Enhancing quality of life by improving your ability to perform daily routines such as walking, carrying groceries, or playing with your children.

But what if you just don't have access to a gym, feel embarrassed about working out surrounded by all those so-called perfect bodies, or you're on a fixed budget?

It's still possible to get a decent full-body workout—including all the benefits of strength training—with no more equipment than a few sets of dumbbells and a good attitude. The following is an example of a twenty-five-minute, full-body workout to do right in your own home. (Remember to consult a physician before beginning any exercise program.)

Crunch (Abdominals): Lie on your back, knees bent and feet flat on the floor, feet and knees together. Place your hands behind your head but don't interlock your fingers. Keep your head and neck relaxed. Movement: Exhale as you contract your abs to bring your shoulders off the floor, hold briefly. Inhale as you slowly lower to starting position. (8 to 10 repetitions)

Lunge (Quadriceps, inner thighs, and glutes): Stand with feet together, hands holding a dumbbell on each hip. Movement: Inhale as you step forward with your right leg and bend your front knee until a ninety-degree angle is formed. Keep your knee directly above your toes during the downward movement to avoid overstressing the knee joint. Exhale as you push off your heel to return to starting position. (8 to 10 repetitions)

Squat (Quadriceps, hamstrings, and glutes): Stand with your feet a little wider than shoulder-width apart. Hold a dumbbell in each hand, arms hanging at your sides. Keep your torso erect and your body weight over your heels. Movement: Inhale as you bend your knees and lower your body as if to sit in a chair until your thighs are as close to parallel to the floor as possible. Do not go lower than this or you will put too much stress on your knees. Exhale as you squeeze your buttocks and come back to the starting position. (8 to 10 repetitions)

Curl (Biceps): Stand with your feet shoulder-width apart, knees relaxed, pelvis tucked, shoulders dropped, and chin level. Hold a dumbbell in each hand, arms extended straight down from your shoulders, palms facing forward. Movement: Exhale as you bend one elbow to bring the dumbbell three-fourths of the way to your shoulder. Inhale as you return to starting position. (8 to 10 repetitions)

Push-ups (Chest, triceps, and shoulders): Start from the up position with your arms almost fully extended, palms flat on the floor and a little more than shoulder-width apart, feet together. Movement: Bend your elbows at a right angle, and then straighten your arms as you exhale while raising your body (if you can't do a standard push-up, instead of balancing off of your toes, try putting your knees on the floor). Keep your back straight by tightening your abdominal muscles. Your body should stay as stiff as possible during the whole movement, and your arms should be the only moving part. (8 to 10 repetitions)

Lateral raises (Shoulders): Hold the dumbbells at your sides with your arms straight. Your knees should be soft and slightly bent, with your chest up and shoulders back. Movement: Raise your arms outward from your sides (keeping your arms straight), moving the dumbbells away from your legs until they are parallel to the ground so that your body forms a letter T, and then lower back down to your side. (8 to 10 repetitions)

One-arm row (Back): Stand with your feet hip-width apart, with your left foot two feet in front of your right. Place your left arm on your left side by your knee, and take your right arm (holding the dumbbell) and let it hang straight down toward the floor. Movement: In one motion, raise your right elbow to your right hip and then back down. Then reverse and do the exercise with your left arm. (8 to 10 repetitions)

Arm extension (Triceps): Lie flat on the floor with your knees bent, hip-width apart. Hold your arms straight up toward the ceiling, holding both dumbbells. Movement: Only bending your elbows (not the upper part of your arms), lower your hands toward your ears, and then back to starting position. (8 to 10 repetitions)

Keep in mind that your muscles adapt to any given exercise, so it's important to increase the level of the weights you are using or vary the method and intensity of the workout to stimulate further strength gains.

So, if you were doing bicep curls using five-pound weights, doing eight repetitions—after about eight weeks, you might be able to perform fifteen repetitions. At this point, you need to either increase the weight or slow down the motion of the exercise to half the speed which would intensify the workout without increasing the weight.

I always believed (and have been following this theory for at least a decade) that in order to build muscle, you have to lift weights at least three to four times per week and complete at least three sets with all your muscle groups. And this doesn't even include doing cardiovascular exercise (i.e., walking, biking, etc.). Lately, however, I've been seeing a lot of hype about getting that super body you've always wanted with a twenty-minute workout only three times per week. Or even better, I know places that promise results with just twenty minutes *once* a week. Are we talking about an oil change here or a workout?

Regardless of the program, when you're trying to build muscles, "the amount of repetitions, sets and the intensity are not as important as taking the muscle to complete exhaustion. That's how you get the best results," says Stephen Rice, MD, PhD, MPH, a sports medicine specialist at the Jersey Shore Medical Center in Neptune, New Jersey.

Working your muscle to fatigue (when you literally can't move another muscle) during exercise actually causes microscopic injuries to the muscle. As the muscle repairs itself, it becomes stronger by building larger fibers to prevent future injury. This is how you sculpt your body. We use weights to help do this because it takes much longer to exhaust the muscles through calisthenics or other types of exercise.

So how will you get the best results from your workout? That depends on your goals and your preferences.

"For some people, a workout needs to be quick or they won't do it at all. Anything is better than nothing!" says C. Jessie Jones, PhD, professor of kinesiology at California State University, Fullerton.

Bottom line: Doing any kind of strength-training regimen is better than not doing it. And yes, just once a week is great for beginners, but you should probably increase to two or three times per week after six months. Keep in mind that you need to increase the weights or vary your workouts about every twelve to fifteen weeks—your muscles need new challenges or they will stop growing. Also, if you're trying to lose weight, remember that larger muscles mean increased strength, improved appearance, and more calories burned. Studies have shown that one pound of muscle burns between thirty to fifty calories per day even when you're not using it—whereas a pound of fat burns only two to five calories per day.

Do It Because It Feels Good—and Make It Automatic

In a study appearing in American College of Sports Medicine's *Health and Fitness Journal*, researchers found that the strongest reason exercisers gave for starting to exercise was that they wanted to achieve fitness. But the investigators also found that feelings were the most powerful motivators for continuing to exercise. What were the top reasons: "Well-being"; "pep and energy"; "enjoyment of activity"; "better sleep"; "more alert and relaxed"; and last was "appearance." They added that although appearance and weight control were extremely important, they weren't the *most* important reasons. Another finding by the researchers was that that those who remained active didn't give much thought to their exercise after the initial planning stages—it became automatic and intrinsic. They also made physical activity a priority in their lives—not that it took over their lives, it just became a priority, like showering in the morning.

And that's something that you can do—on whatever level and in whatever style works for you. Whether it's walking, biking, gardening, or working out at a gym, just make it happen!

▶▶▶▶▶▶▶▶▶▶▶▶▶▶▶▶▶▶▶▶▶▶ PART 2

Empower, Not Willpower

"One person with a belief is equal to a force of 99 who have only interests." —John Stuart Mill

"You've got to find the force inside you." —Joseph Campbell

I'm often asked for the single biggest reason people don't succeed at losing and controlling their weight: I can honestly say that it's all about discipline and willpower. I know. You think I mean *the lack of those qualities*—but no. I mean the opposite: People try to use discipline and willpower to make changes in behavior that really require *empowerment*.

Discipline and willpower will fail you every time. Why is that? Well, I don't know about you, but I'm weak, and when a doughnut is staring me in the face, willpower just doesn't cut it. Sure, I might walk away from that doughnut or push it away once or twice, but honestly, there's only so long I can tell myself not to eat something I know for a fact tastes great. Come on now, we have to stop kidding ourselves. We need something a bit more powerful than willpower to battle Krispy Kreme kryptonite!

There's a huge difference between being empowered to make changes and simply relying on your own willpower. Just to illustrate the contrast, take a look at the definitions. Empower means to invest with power or to equip or supply with an *ability*, whereas willpower involves having strength or control. Clearly, giving yourself the power and ability to achieve something *provides the energy you need to reach your goals.*

In the following four Steps I'll be giving you all the empowerment strategies you need to implement the tools you've already acquired so that they do truly become second nature. No longer will you have to depend on something as weak and undependable as willpower to meet your weight-loss goals. Instead, your efforts will be fueled by the far more potent energy that comes from feeling truly empowered.

Excuse Busting

"People are always blaming their circumstances for what they are. I don't believe in circumstances. The people who get on in the world are the people who get up and look for the circumstances they want, and if they can't find them, make them." —George Bernard Shaw

"Ninety-nine percent of the failures come from people who have the habit of making excuses." —George Washington Carver

I was sitting at a restaurant with my wife, having just finished a plate of tiramisu. I don't normally eat tiramisu, or any dessert for that matter, but tonight was different. We were recently married and had started to eat out more often. For a while, I had done well with thinking ahead about menu choices and sticking to a livable diet, even though eating out happens to be one of my Diet Busters. But that evening, when the waiter asked if we wanted dessert, I asked my wife if she'd like to split a tiramisu. What's one dessert, after all, or even better, a split dessert?

The only thing was, I'd been having more and more "just one" desserts as I ate out more often. And I was getting lax in other areas as well—eating more bread before the meal and ordering more high-calorie foods. As a result, I'd noticed that I'd started to gain a few pounds. After a while, I actually started to get annoyed. Not at myself, but at my wife. I mean, if I weren't married and she didn't like eating out, I wouldn't be getting fat again, right?

Wrong. In fact, my wife had absolutely nothing to do with my weight gain. I realized that I was blaming her and using her as the *excuse* for my weight gain—and *my* choices to nibble. So I talked to my wife, and we came up with a number of restaurants we both enjoyed that served a healthier menu. I went back to planning what I was going to eat beforehand, and we agreed to ask that the waitperson not put the bread basket on the table. We also began to ask for the check when we ordered our coffee and declined to see the dessert menu to avoid temptation.

Who Are We Kidding?

Why was I blaming my wife, anyway? Who did I think I was kidding? My wife wasn't even the one who'd suggested we order the tiramisu—that was me, too. If anyone should know that one is always responsible for one's food choices, it's me. "Taking responsibility" is my mantra. I refer to it as "the unwanted stepchild of dieting."

Client interviews as well as research show that the vast majority of successful losers attribute their ability to maintain weight loss to their understanding that they are the *only* ones responsible for their weight control. While that may sound like bad news to begin with, once you understand that *you* are responsible for your weight—and that it's a choice *you* are making—well, it's exhilarating, because *it means you have the power to change.*

For instance, take a look at Helen. She had three children ages eight, twelve, and fourteen, and she worked part-time at hospital. Helen was a very busy woman. If you were to ask her about dieting, her answer might have sounded something like this: "Who has time to lose weight—between getting breakfast on the table, getting the kids off to school, running errands, work, the day never ends. *I wish I could hire someone to lose the weight for me!*"

Helen was typical of many people who have too many responsibilities and too little time. She was swamped with everyday life, and the mere thought of having to actually do something about her weight seemed overwhelming. Not only that, but according to Helen, she was "cursed with bad genes." Both her mother and father were overweight, and she just knew that she was destined for the same uncomfortable path.

By the time Helen was in her forties, she was completely inactive, had gained a few more pounds, and had tried every diet in the book without success. She blamed her busy schedule, bad genes, and lack of willpower for her weight problem, her inactivity, and her discomfort.

Was Helen responsible for the "bad genes" that had given her a slow metabolism? No. What about her busy schedule and responsibilities? Well, she certainly couldn't shirk her obligations to her family, work, and social life. So how was Helen to be held responsible for gaining those fifty-five-plus pounds?

The fact is that Helen, whatever her biology and lifestyle, may not have been responsible for everything that made her overweight, but she was responsible for how she *responded* to the circumstances surrounding her life, which include her eating habits and lack of physical activity.

Dr. Barry Schlenker, PhD, a professor of psychology at the University of Florida, reporting in *Research in Organizational Behavior* explained responsibility as "the psychological glue that attaches an individual to an event and to the prescriptions governing it." That doesn't mean other people, circumstances, or events can't have a profound influence on how we think, feel, or act, it just means that they shouldn't be *blamed* for the way we respond to them.

The Blame Game

Much as we may acknowledge and understand that, in the end, blame isn't going to get us anywhere, we all, nevertheless, fall prey to its charms at one time or another. In fact, I don't know what we would do without blame. One might argue that it's the cornerstone of our psychological makeup. Blame is the comfortable path to take when you want to avoid issues that move you toward your goals. Blame lets you sidestep responsibility for a while—it's what I call "antiresponsible" behavior. Blame is responsibility's arch-enemy, and it needs to be handled aggressively.

Don't get me wrong. Blame can be wonderful, in the short run. It allows you to avoid taking a necessary action—it gets you off the hook from acting responsibly. Blame is an easy out. In terms of diet, it helps you to not focus on your own weight-control efforts while you concentrate on all the reasons you've given yourself for why it's out of your hands. But, in the end, blame is just a short-term strategy for getting yourself off the hook, even making you feel better. Long-term, it just doesn't work.

Believe me, when it comes to blame, I'm an expert. I really understand its ins and outs. For years, I was a master of the art of blaming, but it worked to my disadvantage. Blaming other people or external circumstances, situations, or events is just a way to excuse ourselves from doing what we really know we need to do, and once I understood that, I was able to find the tools I needed to quit the blame game and bust the excuses I'd been making. And those are exactly the tools I'm going to be sharing with you. But first, let's take a closer look at the two faces of blame so that you'll be able to recognize it easily when you see it in yourself.

The Two Faces of Blame

You can "externalize" blame by placing it outside yourself—in other people (e.g., "How can I lose weight when I have an unsupportive family?"), situations, or circumstances (e.g., "I inherited bad genes." "I don't have time to plan healthy, low-calorie meals. I'm just too busy." "I have to keep all those sugary foods in the house for the kids"). Or you can "internalize" it by blaming yourself (e.g., "I'm a weak person." "I don't have the strength or the willpower to stick to my plan").

Externalizing Blame Behavior

One of the classic blaming explanations for externalizers is making "bad genes" the culprit for their weight problem. Is having "bad genes" a valid argument?

Well, we've already discussed the Pima Indians and seen how they overcame "bad" genes, so we know it's possible to stabilize weight by making the right choices. Nevertheless, since the fifties, researchers have argued that many aspects of personality and temperament are inborn. Some babies are just born more or less intense, outgoing, whiny, adventurous, timid, somber, persistent, or expressive—you name the trait.

So where does this take you?

Doesn't a bad gene pool absolve you of responsibility for being overweight? Of course, there are people who insist that biology both explains and excuses all good and bad behavior. But I would argue that knowing as much as possible about your biology (and family history) leads to an entirely different conclusion: You can use the knowledge you have and be responsible for making it work *for* you.

Having access to information such as a predisposition to obesity or diabetes is an immensely useful tool in your quest for self-knowledge. It would be foolish to ignore *anything* that helps you to know yourself more fully and avoid the potential booby traps in your life. But this knowledge is not a life sentence—it's a way to improve your life. It gives you a personal barometer for determining what to avoid and what to embrace. It helps you chart a smarter course.

Internalizing Blame Behavior

Too often, internalizers define themselves as hopeless or lost before they begin. They use phrases such as, "I can't do it, so why try?" "I'm no good at that." "It's all my fault." "I wish I were never born." And when they examine their experiences and failures, their reasoning follows a similarly self-defeating line of reasoning: "Why am I fat? Because I'm weak and have no discipline, no self-control, no willpower." When an internalizer fails at a diet, he or she figures, "I'm just not the sort of person who deserves to be in good shape, so I might as well get used to it."

What internalizers don't seem to understand is that *being responsible* is a very different thing from blaming oneself. Taking responsibility means being accountable to yourself. Self-blame means believing that everything is your fault. The first is empowering and propels you forward, the second is counter-productive, depressing, and a futile exercise in beating yourself up. Remember: Blaming yourself is as destructive as blaming someone or something else for your own misguided efforts.

When you *in*ternalize, you suppress and swallow your frustrations, heaping the blame on yourself without attempting to examine why you have not achieved your goal or trying to discover what it is you can do to correct the problem. Self-blame damages your self-esteem and self-efficacy, and destroys any possible motivation you might have had to act. And because having a strong sense of self-esteem and self-efficacy are critical components of successful weight control, the blame works against you and takes you further away from your weight-loss goal.

A number of years ago, I read an interview in *Esquire* magazine with the famous exercise guru Jack LaLanne, who, I believe, perfectly summed up the nature of excuses and responsibility:

"Do you know there's more fat people than there's ever been in our history?" Jack said. "It's terrible. People who don't eat right, don't exercise. They drink, then go to church, and then it's 'Dear God, dear God! Please help me with this. Please give me that!' Hey, God is not going to do a thing for you. You do it. He gives you the power to do it.

Listen, in the sixty-eight years I've been doing this, I've never once heard Jesus knocking on my door at five in the morning, saying, 'Jack, I'll work out for you today.' "

Don't Turn Away from Helping Yourself

▶ Be aware of who or what has come to offer help and advice—and take it, once you know its purpose is to help you improve yourself

▶ Taking responsibility means seizing those golden moments when you are given a gift of knowledge, of life, or of opportunity

▶ Do not allow ideas of predetermination to stop you from pursuing your goals

A perfect example of blame: A Harris Interactive poll conducted for *The Wall Street Journal* online health-industry edition found that 89 percent of those polled said TV commercials were to blame for people eating and drinking more than was good for them. The fact is, there is no one more responsible than you for the way your life works out. You have choices despite the impact other people or circumstances have on how you think, feel, or act. Starting with your parents, other people *will* affect you in great and small ways. Keep in mind, however, that one of the key characteristics of *all* successful weight losers is their ability to avoid blaming and accept responsibility for whatever failures or setbacks trip them up along the road to dieting bliss.

Blaming means that it's not within your power or control to fix the problem. No successful person would ever buy into the belief that his or her life was not within his control and that all he could do was surrender to the whims of chance.

If you're going to be successful in managing your weight, as I know you can be, it's time to stop playing the blame game. Here's one powerful weapon you can use to combat the insidious incursion of blame.

Use the Power of Language

Altering the language you use to tell your story and express your frustrations can help you change. Language shapes the way you view things, just as your view of things shapes the way you talk about them. It follows, therefore, that the words you use can influence the way you think.

You need to listen to what you're saying when you're thinking or talking about yourself. If you find that you're making yourself the object of other people's actions (e.g., "If Harry hadn't taken me to that Italian restaurant, I wouldn't have been tempted to eat all that pasta") or of circumstances (e.g., "My parents really saddled me with terrible obesity genes"), what you need to do is turn those sentences around so that you become the *subject,* the primary actor and cause of whatever it is that's happening in your world. One way you can do that is by beginning your sentences with the word *I.* Many mental health professionals suggest that by using *I* statements when discussing issues, you can affirmatively transform your behavior. For instance: "I know that I often overeat when I'm in this situation." Or, "I tend to [fill in the blank] when the going gets rough." You don't want to use a dead-end statement (i.e., internalizing) like, "If Jenny hadn't been in my life, I wouldn't be fifty pounds overweight." State specifically what *you* may be doing wrong so that *you* can correct it instead of blaming yourself or other people.

Think of something you did today that connects with unhealthy eating habits. Describe it by beginning your sentence with the word *I.* Follow that with an action verb to show that you did something or are doing something. Don't use any form of the verb "to be" such as "I am," which would be to describe yourself in passive terms.

Here's an example. One of the excuses I hear all the time is, "I am really busy, and don't have the time to pay attention to the nutrient information of everything I put into my mouth." Yes, you may be very busy, but you are doing yourself a disservice by offering this up as a reason for not eating properly.

Almost everybody these days lives a hectic lifestyle, but is that the real reason for your food choices? Busy people need to prioritize, especially when it comes to getting healthy by losing excess weight, so the truth of the situation might be closer to: "I'm very busy, and I make choices every minute of every day, and right now, reviewing what I eat every day does *not* take priority over other matters in my life." That statement is honest and candid and lets you see that you can *choose* to make a change.

When you put the word *me* at the end of your sentence rather than *I* at the beginning, you confirm your passivity and helplessness and allow whatever negative pattern you're following to continue. Think what a difference it makes when you change, "My boss is making life hell for me, which is why I'm always into the bags of chips when I get home" to "I choose to stay in this job despite the fact that my boss undermines my authority. I respond to this stress by coming home and eating unhealthy foods to make myself feel better." Or changing "My husband is always picking fights with me, which forces me to overeat junk food" to "My husband and I argue, so I respond angrily, get stressed out, and do myself harm by bingeing on junk food." In both instances, the first statement keeps you a victim. The second opens up a whole new line of inquiry and potential action by giving you the opportunity to ask yourself, "Why do I choose to eat junk food in stressful situations? What can I do to change that?"

Doing that is taking a positive step toward developing a new pattern of individual responsibility.

To get started, get out your notebook and write down *five* situations, events, or circumstances that did not go according to plan in terms of weight loss—whether or not you think they were your fault. Now go back and read through each one. When you get to the part about what went wrong or where the problem occurred and how it affected what and how you ate or your physical activity, rephrase it so that *you're* the one who is ultimately responsible. Don't place any blame on another person, luck, connections, or yourself. Blame is easy to recognize because it most often manifests itself in excuse-making—the antithesis of accepting responsibility.

1...2...3...4...5...

The Truth About Excuses

A doctor has a stethoscope, a gardener has a lawnmower, a plumber has a plunger, and a blamer has excuses. Excuses are the tools for the blamer to use in order to avoid responsibility. "Excuses have the paradoxical quality of being widely condemned but widely employed," says Beth A. Pontari, PhD, in the *Journal of Social and Clinical Psychology*. You, too, have probably come up with hundreds of clever excuses for not reaching your weight goal. As reported in *Personality and Social Psychology Review*,

Excuses are self-serving explanations, or accounts that aim to reduce personal responsibility for questionable events, thereby disengaging core components of the self from the incident. Their goal is to convince audiences, often the actor included, that a questionable event is not as much the actor's fault as it might otherwise appear to be; and to the extent that the actor is at fault, the incident is portrayed as springing from less central rather than more central aspects of self (e.g., carelessness rather than stupidity).

Some of the most common excuses for not succeeding with one's weight-loss goals are:

▸ "I'm big boned"

▸ "I have a slow metabolism"

▸ "I don't have enough money to join a gym"

▸ "I have to work and my schedule is just too tight to exercise"

▸ "I have three kids, a husband, a dog, and in-laws who live two houses away from me—I'm a busy woman"

▸ "Not sure what's wrong with my body. I just have *bad genes,* and can't lose weight no matter how hard I try"

▸ "I'm too tired to think about what I can and can't eat"

▸ "It's too late for me"

▸ "I don't have enough time to follow a diet"

▸ "I work in a bakery/restaurant/candy factory, and the stuff's all around me, either for free or discounted. I can't change my job just to lose weight"

▸ "I don't know where to begin"

▸ "It's just too hard"

▸ "I'm afraid I'm going to hurt my bad knee if I start walking more"

▸ "I'm too self-conscious about the way I look to be more active"

▸ "Every time I mention wanting to get more exercise my family and friends discourage me"

▸ "I can't get anyone to watch my kids"

▸ "No one I know does any exercise"

▸ "The air in my area is polluted"

▸ "I just can't get motivated—it doesn't excite me"

▸ "People will have to like me the way I am. I don't judge people by how skinny they are."

When you blame, you're excusing yourself from responsibility.

The trouble is, some excuses appear so airtight that you can talk yourself out of doing what you know you have to do. In fact, excuses work (just like blame works), according to C. R. Snyder, PhD, a professor of psychology at the University of Kansas. They help to distance you from the uncomfortable consequences of failure; they insulate you from potential damage to your self-esteem; they help you maintain a sense of control because you shift responsibility, which means you never lost control of the situation. But, just like blame, excuses can lead to unpleasant outcomes—such as being overweight. Dr. Schlenker clarifies this by saying, "Excuses are designed to minimize responsibility and thereby disengage the self from the event. If the event is nonrecurring (e.g., a rare task failure or rule violation) or trivial (e.g., failure in an unimportant domain or violation of a petty rule), disengagement of self poses many advantages and few disadvantages. However, if the event is recurring or important, disengagement through excuses produces problems if responsibility is also undermined for future performances." And knowing that you think losing weight is important, disengaging from responsibility for your weight by making excuses is clearly problematic.

Excuses Are Not Reasons

When I was overweight, I, too, cushioned myself with excuses until I finally wised up and figured out that I was just fooling myself. That was when I realized that by focusing on *reasons* rather than *excuses*, I'd be taking a giant step toward accepting responsibility for myself and my weight.

Excuses are merely vehicles of blame, attempts to rationalize away responsibility for why things didn't go the way you wanted them. Reasons are something quite different. Through reflection, assessment, and analysis (using the detective work I've been teaching you throughout this book), you can identify what you *did* or *didn't do* that caused you to be unsuccessful in the past—these are your reasons. Discovering those reasons is how you learn.

What I'm going to do now is give you a *reason* to stop the rationalizing and find an Excuse Buster instead.

What's an Excuse Buster?

An Excuse Buster is a persuasive self-talk argument made to counteract your justification (aka excuse) for not controlling your weight. When you practice Excuse Busting, you think up positive strategies that replace negative excuses. As we've already discussed, there are many things in life (such as brushing your teeth) that you do automatically, without having to think about whether or not you're going to do them. Creating a process of automatic, "pre–thought-out" answers to counteract our most common excuses can help us to banish them once and for all.

Think of this as a battle. Excuses are the enemy. They're what may be preventing you from losing weight and keeping it off. So, you have to be relentless when you go into combat against them and work out your Plan of Attack. This formula will help you develop a winning strategy.

1. **Get to Know Your Enemy:** Knowledge is power! What obstacles do you face? What are the excuses that keep you from losing weight?
2. **Fire Back:** Have your ammunition ready! Develop Excuse Busters that help shoot down even your strongest excuses.
3. **Outsmart Your Enemy:** Even if your Excuse Busters don't work, you're unstoppable with a Plan B!

Get to Know Your Enemy

First, take the time to think about which of your weight-loss goals it's been the most difficult for you to achieve. Which of them do you most often find excuses to avoid? For example, here's a goal that Sue, one of my clients, was struggling with:

"I'm having a hard time curbing my nighttime eating. I always have really good intentions to stop, but when 10 PM rolls around, for one reason or another, I always end up stuffing my face with snacks. There goes my goal to not eat after dinner."

Which of your goals have been the most difficult for you to reach? List *five* in your notebook.

1 . . . 2 . . . 3 . . . 4 . . . 5 . . .

Notice that Sue chose to remove herself from the situation and put the reason out there in the ether—"for one reason or another"—as if she had nothing to do with it. When we talked about the actual *reasons* why she was eating at night, Sue said, "I was so careful about not eating too much at dinner that I was just ravenous by the time ten o'clock rolled around." Remember: There are plenty of excuses, but there are *no good reasons* for not achieving your weight-loss goals.

When she was finally determined to recognize the excuses she was making for her poor choices, and why she ended up snacking every evening, she told me, "I would always find myself trying to justify my eating by saying, 'It's okay just this once' or 'This little snack doesn't make that much of a difference.' Until, I started thinking about it, it didn't even occur to me what I was doing!"

Now, it's your turn. Remember, knowledge is power! Take the time to brainstorm all the excuses you can think of to get out of working toward each one of the *five* problem goals you identified above. Include all your self-doubts, fears, and insecurities because, yes, those are excuses, too. Be creative! Challenge yourself! Knowing your excuses will give you the power to fight them.

1 . . . 2 . . . 3 . . . 4 . . . 5 . . .

Fire Back

To defuse your excuses forever, you need to come up with persuasive arguments to counteract your most common justifications for not getting things done. If your excuses have no power, you won't use them.

My recommendation is that you begin with a little self-talk on the subject. Look at the excuses you just brainstormed. How might you fight back against each one? The key is to have a powerful, ready-made Excuse Buster. These six examples will give you an idea of how to proceed for yourself:

Excuse: I only live once. Why diet?

Excuse Buster: I may only live once, but if I'm not happy during that life, and if I get sick because of the complications of being overweight, I'm not taking very good care of myself. If I only live once, I'm going to do my best to make it great.

Excuse: I'm genetically made this way. Everyone in my family has a big gut or backside.

Excuse Buster: I may be genetically inclined to gain weight easily in my midsection/backside, but I know I can control how much weight I do or do not gain. I can break my most destructive eating patterns and learn new patterns to combat my genetic predispositions. Plus, it can't be just a coincidence that everyone in my family is chronically inactive in addition to being chronically overweight!

Excuse: I've lost weight before and couldn't keep it off, so what's the point?

Excuse Buster: Trying and failing is not a valid reason for not giving weight loss another chance. I know I can lose twenty pounds because I've done it before, and this time I will do everything I need to do to keep the weight off. I won't give in or give up.

Excuse: I have a standing dinner date with my best friends on Wednesdays, and I have Sunday dinner at my parents' house. Talk about temptation! I go through half a loaf of buttery garlic bread and some heavy meat dish one day, and too much barbecue and dessert the next. What else can I do? I'm not doing the cooking and there's nothing else to eat!

Excuse Buster: In the future, I'll explain my dietary restrictions to my friends and my parents. I'll plan in advance what I'm going to eat in the restaurant with my friends and ask them to support me. I'll offer to either cook or bring my own meal to my parents' house if it's inconvenient for them to make what I can eat. I'll also be sure to have a light snack beforehand so I'm not tempted to go overboard. I won't take the bait if they tease me or tempt me.

Excuse: I'll eat it just this one time. . . . Or I just want it because I want it, and it's only one time, so what's the big deal?

Excuse Buster: Life is made up of many "one times," so I'd better stop fooling myself. I have to decide what I want in life and make it happen for myself. I realize that losing weight is about free choice. *I* decided that *my* choice was to lose weight. I was the one who made that decision, and I want to stick to it. My health and self-confidence aren't worth the extra calories in "just this one time." Plus, as the saying goes, "Nothing tastes as good as skinny feels!"

Now it's your turn.

Take out your notebook and think of at least *five* Excuses and the Excuse Busters that match them.

Excuse: _____

Excuse Busters: _____

When you're done writing them out, keep the pages handy. For example, post them on the fridge or make them mobile—keep them folded and in your back pocket, handbag, knapsack, or briefcase. Remember, forgetting your Excuse Buster is not a valid excuse!

Make an Excuse Buster "Piggy Bank"

When it comes to sticking with your weight-loss goals, having powerful Excuse Busters handy is like having money in the bank. So why not "bank" them. Write out each of the Excuse Busters you've come up with for each of your excuses and put them in separate jars or bowls—one for each excuse. Then, when you hear yourself making that excuse, you can pull one out—like having cash on hand when you need it.

Outsmart Your Enemy with a Plan B

To make Excuse Busting airtight, you'll also need to have a backup plan, or what I call a Plan B. It may happen that you run into an excuse that is stubbornly immune to all your best Excuse Busters. Then it's time for the Plan B you've come up with to kick in. Your Plan B must be as effective as Plan A. It must be just as compatible with reaching your weight-loss goals, and it must be ready in advance. Again, once your plans are in place, they'll become automatic and you won't even have to think about them. For example, your excuse is that you don't have time to exercise. Your Excuse Buster is that you can run in your own neighborhood early in the morning (Plan A), but it's raining and you don't want to get soaked. In that case, your Plan B could be to go to an aerobics class, use a track at the gym, or play an exercise videotape in your own home. This type of proactive behavior guarantees that you won't leave too many circumstances (like the weather) to chance and really helps to accomplish your goals.

Another Plan B: "I frequently snack at night because I'm worried about work the next day." Your Excuse Buster is that you'll eliminate all potentially unhealthy snacks from your home so you only have healthy snacks on hand (Plan A). But your kids keep bringing home chips and other fattening snack foods even though you've asked them not to. Your Plan B might be to have a baggie filled with special low-calorie treats that you have only when you're tempted by stuff the kids have brought in. Or you might want to put your foot down and impress upon them that you're not going to tolerate junk food in the house because it's simply not healthy. Remember, you'll never achieve your goal, no matter how badly you might want it, if you let yourself coast on excuses. Make your own choices, not excuses, and don't let outside circumstances make choices for you. Excuse Busting, however, is not an exact science. Every now and then you'll come up against an excuse that is, well, actually justified. If, for example, you're injured and can't run, there really isn't any way to talk your way out of the problem. But those are exactly the times when you need a Plan B—or even a Plan C. If you can't run, maybe you can swim. Is there a public pool you could use? Or perhaps you could do some upper-body strength training at home. Developing these alternative Excuse Busters in advance is an indication that you are consciously choosing to lose weight.

Take a look at the examples below, then develop your own list of *unbustable,* airtight excuses, and build up an arsenal of your own Plan Bs.

Unbustable Excuse: I have to work late to finish a project and can't go to the gym.

Plan B: I will go for a long walk after lunch on days when I might have to work late. Or, I will get up extra early and bike to work. I will bring an extra set of dumbbells to the office, and on those days I have to work late I'll use an empty conference room or office and do some weight training. Even if it's only for twenty minutes, that's still better than nothing.

Unbustable Excuse: I'm traveling in an area where there are only fast-food places to eat—it's hard to eat healthily.

Plan B: I will investigate various fast-food restaurants in advance and try to find out what I can eat at each one to ensure that I stay on my weight-loss program. I will go to a supermarket to stock up on healthy snacks to take with me before I get on the road so that I don't become ravenous and end up pulling off the road to eat two Big Macs.

Now it's your turn to review each one of your excuses and Excuse Busters, then try to think of any obstacles or setbacks that might make your excuse *unbustable* and come up with a Plan B. Write your Plan Bs in your notebook, where they'll be ready when you need them.

Excuse: _____

Excuse Buster: _____

Plan B: _____

Energize Your Choice

I know you understand that you're as responsible for your weight as you are for every other aspect of your life, and I know you've made the choice to lose weight and keep it off by creating your own livable diet. But I also know, as I've already said, that no one is perfect, and that you'll have your diet-busting moments just as I did when I ordered that tiramisu. The tools I've provided in this Step, along with the ones you'll be learning in the Steps that follow, are all designed to provide you with the power you need to see your choice through to your goal and to keep you on track in those unavoidable moments of weakness when you want to blame someone else or make excuses for not sticking with your plan. Consider them weapons in your weight-loss arsenal, and know that the more weapons you have, the better armed you'll be whenever temptation rears its ugly head.

Craft a Strategy

"The secret of getting ahead is getting started. The secret of getting started is breaking your complex, overwhelming tasks into small manageable tasks, and then starting on the first one." —Mark Twain

Whether you're planning a major, military offensive or playing a game of chess, if you're going to be a winner, you need to have a strategy—you need to think ahead, know what your next move is going to be, and then the move after that. If you don't know how you're going to achieve your victory, you're likely to be blindsided, sidetracked, or knocked out of the game. In other words, you need not only to have a long term goal—taking the fort from the enemy or your opponent's queen—but also a well thought-out strategy for how you're going to do that.

I know, and you know, what your long-term goal is—losing weight and keeping it off—but until you have a well thought-out strategy for doing that—for taking the steps that will get you there—it's probably not much more likely to happen than I am to win a gold medal in ski-jumping at the next winter Olympics (and just so we're clear, I ski maybe once every five years). I suppose it could happen, but the odds are not in my favor. And I'm assuming that one of the reasons you're reading this book is that you'd like to leave less up to chance and shift those odds in your favor.

I'm sure you've already resolved to lose weight (and how many New Year's resolutions have you made and broken in the past?), but chances are that just isn't going to cut it. Of course, you may win the weight-loss lottery, but according to the *Journal of the American Dietetic Association,* those individuals who used goal setting and goal-attainment skills enhanced their chance of "making and maintaining improvements in nutrition-related behaviors" by 84 percent.

But why should that surprise you? Most of what you do in life probably requires some degree of strategic planning, even if it's figuring out the best route from the dry cleaner to the post office to the supermarket when you set out to do errands. We have no problem coming up with detailed strategies when we're planning an event like a wedding. In fact, we obsess over every last detail—the band, location, dress, tux, and caterer. But when it comes to our weight, yes, we may think about it, but we don't give it a fraction of the *strategic passion* it deserves.

If you've ever taken a long road trip with your family you probably didn't just hop in the car and turn the key without doing a fair amount of preparation in advance. You probably looked at a map, purchased a guide book or two, peeked at a few Web sites, decided how many days the trip would take, how far you could travel each day, where you'd be staying each night, and even planned some great, exciting side trips along the way to keep you motivated and excited.

You might have arrived at your destination without doing that, but chances are you'd have made a few wrong turns and maybe even found yourself traveling in circles for a while. Well, you've probably been traveling in circles long enough on the road to permanent weight loss, so isn't it time to make sure you get where you want to go?

You already have all the tools you need, from discovering your Fat Patterns and Diet Traps to finding Calorie Bargains, creating a safe, personal food environment, and increasing your physical activity. You've quit making excuses and you're ready to get going. So your job now is to craft a good strategy for using those tools to your best advantage. Here's what you're going to do:

▸ You'll systematically learn how to reach your goal weight by plotting out the detailed steps, and writing them all down

▸ To be most effective, you won't simply say, "I'm going to lose twenty-five pounds." You will devise a kind of roadmap, complete with contingencies for possible obstacles and detours. Then you'll track your progress consistently and thoughtfully

▸ You'll not only plan what to eat, but how you will deal with foods you find irresistible

▸ You will make a plan for weaving physical activity into your schedule

▸ Most of all, you will create a strategy for dealing with your most slip-prone temptations and situations.

Could you achieve your goals without this kind of strategic planning? Of course you could! You could also win the lottery. But, again, it's unlikely. Most of the time, achieving and maintaining weight loss does not happen by accident.

Goals in the Context of the Rest of Your Life

You don't live in a vacuum. Your actions and decisions affect your loved ones to one degree or another. Even those of you who are single have family, coworkers, and friends who are affected by your actions. So, when setting a goal, you need to take these relationships into account by asking questions such as:

▸ How does this goal affect my family?
▸ How does this goal affect my responsibilities at work?
▸ How does this goal affect my friends and coworkers?
▸ How does this goal relate to the other activities in my life?
▸ Will I need to give up some activities to make room for it?
▸ How does it relate to my community or environment?

If you sense that the pursuit of your goal is creating friction with other people, you need to confront this issue head-on before proceeding. Discuss your goals with your loved ones. More than likely they'll be pleased that you've decided to make a positive change. If they have any worries, you can assure them that you know what you're doing. For example, let's say you're married and decide to train for an upcoming 10K run. In all likelihood, your spouse will be thrilled for you and happy to see you in great physical shape. But he or she might also be concerned that such training will take away from some valuable family time. To take such concerns into account, you might suggest that your spouse do some of parts of the activity with you, or you could offer to cut down on other solitary activities, like watching TV or doing the crossword puzzle, and use that time to prepare for the 10K.

You should also keep in mind, however, that any serious goal cannot be conditional. When I hear people couch their aspirations in what I call "If/then statements," I immediately question the seriousness of their intent. Examples of this include: "If I just get my career on track, then I'll finally be able to focus on losing weight." Or: "If I had a gym near my house, then I could really start getting in shape." The problem with these statements is that they don't provide momentum or motivation for long-term goals; on the contrary, they allow momentum to fizzle. Postponing the pursuit of a goal makes it seem less serious, less urgently desired.

You may not be able to reach a goal right away, but you can begin taking serious steps toward it. Do not bide your time waiting for the right moment to hit. Patience is important, but don't be so patient that you sit back and wait for a sign that the perfect conditions are opening up, which, after all, may never occur.

Get SMARTER

"The Truth About Dieting," a major survey published by *Consumer Reports* in June 2002, reported that most people succeed at weight loss "by conscious effort." And "83 percent of all successful losers said they lost weight entirely on their own." What this means for you is what I've been saying all along. The key to weight loss is not to adhere to someone else's program, but to create your own plan, make it a priority on *your* personal to-do list, and get SMARTER about how you're going to make it happen.

There are essentially seven characteristics of effective, strategic planning and goal setting that you can remember with the easy acronym SMARTER:

▸ **S**pecific

▸ **M**otivating

▸ **A**chievable

▸ **R**ewarding

▸ **T**actical

▸ **E**valuated

▸ **R**evisable

Specific

Jonathan is a forty-nine-year-old software engineer working in Boston. He works hard, has a large family, and enjoys the occasional golf game, but lately his game has been suffering because he is significantly overweight. He can't move on the golf course without becoming winded, and his doctor has advised that he lose weight because his father died of heart disease–related complications. In talking with me, Jonathan mentioned that he had a "very clear and precise goal—to lose weight."

Well, that's certainly an admirable goal, but it's not very "clear and precise." Saying you want to lose weight is a beginning, but if you think it ends there, you're mistaken. When determining your goals and coming up with any strategy, you need to make them *specific* and *measurable*. What does that mean? It means that instead of simply making a vague statement such as "I'm going to lose weight," Jonathan (or you) might say, "I'm going to lose forty-five pounds in a year." In fact, the *Journal of Sports Science* has reported that any time an individual assigns specific goals for themselves, they achieve a better performance than when goals are nonspecific. The investigators also noted that as you increase realistic specificity (e.g., twenty pounds in sixteen weeks vs. twenty pounds) you increase your performance. And a study in *Perceptual and Motor Skills* also reports that having specific, clear goals can reduce the level of effort required to attain them as well as your level of stress.

Goals should answer the questions *how, when, where,* and *why,* and should help to set your course of action. So, for example, Jonathan needed not only to make his ultimate goal more specific—such as "I want to lose forty-five pounds in a year," he also needed to determine what he would have to do each day to reach that goal. For example, to lose forty-five pounds in a year, he would have to cut 157,500 calories from his current eating program and/or increase his physical activity. That would break down to about 3000 calories per week, or about 428 calories per day. Once he'd figured that out, Jonathan would have not only a clear and specific long-term goal (to lose forty-five pounds in a year), but also equally clear mid-term (cut out 3000 calories a week) and short-term (cut out 428 calories a day) goals.

We'll be talking more about mid- and short-term goals in the pages that follow. For now, here are some additional examples of specific, clear, and precise *overall* or *long-term* goals:

▶ Decrease my waist size from a forty to a thirty-four in forty-eight weeks

▶ Lose fifty pounds in one hundred weeks

▶ Walk every morning at 10 AM around the lake near home for a to-tal of ten miles walked per week

▶ Run my first 5K race thirty-six weeks from now.

So you see how goals can vary, but that doesn't matter as long as they are as specific as possible.

Motivating

My clients say some amazing things when they talk about what they're going to do to lose weight. I hear things like, "I'm going to start running every single morning at 6 AM—you just wait and see! I'm going to get rid of these forty pounds once and for all." Of course, that sounds great, but the reality is that the guy who said it never gets out of bed before 8 AM. Plus, he *hates* running. How does he think he can stick to a change or lifestyle adjustment he hates? Sometimes we actually make these extreme plans just *because* we know we'll never be able to stick with them and we're giving ourselves an excuse for weaseling out of our commitment. But that, of course, is just another form of self-sabotage.

Then there's Janice, from Reno, Nevada, who thought it would be great to start eating the low-calorie foods she saw in the supermarket.

She stocked her fridge with every frozen, diet entrée she could get her hands on. She would just force herself to eat them for lunch and dinner— at least that was her plan. Most people do enjoy these meals, and, as I've said, they can be a simple way to avoid overeating because the portion size is already controlled and they are quick to prepare. But they just didn't satisfy Janice. She never got used to them and eating them didn't become automatic. After about a month, she was off her low-calorie, frozen-food diet for good.

Clearly, setting a goal you hate is not going to keep you motivated for very long. You'll greatly improve your chances of success when you enjoy the *process* of working toward accomplishment, not just the end result. When a curious infant picks up objects and examines them, tastes them, and throws them around, he or she is learning, not because of any outside reward, but for the pleasure of learning itself. Later on, children who enjoy learning for learning's sake, not just for reaping good grades or pleasing their parents, are happier and better students.

Here's another classic example of someone who needed to find a more motivating goal. Jennifer wanted to lose weight and start exercising for health reasons, but she really thought exercise was silly. "Why do something like jog around the neighborhood?" she commented. "It doesn't get me anywhere and it just wastes my time."

If she were to force herself to jog around the neighborhood, she'd be unlikely to sustain her goal. She'd be bored and resent wasting her time. What she needed to do was find a physical activity she considered enjoyable as well as useful and functional, not just exercising for the sake of exercising. That might be walking or riding her bicycle to work. In either case, she'd be getting somewhere she needed to go, and, at the same time, she'd be saving gas money and helping the environment by creating less pollution. Or, she might take up gardening. Growing her own food would be a healthy alternative, she'd be saving on her supermarket bills, and she'd be out in the fresh air. In addition to being intrinsically enjoyable, however, a goal, to be truly motivating, also has to be somewhat of a challenge. Just switching from regular to diet soda, for example, might help you to lose weight, but it isn't much of a goal.

As a rule of thumb, if you set a goal that's too easy to reach, you stand the chance of losing interest in pursuing it—as you might with any conquest that seems too easy. So try not to underestimate yourself or what you are capable of doing.

A true goal requires you to marshal your energy, resources, and skills, and really focus. It requires a higher level of performance than you may have imagined you had in you. It gives you a higher occasion to rise to, as well as a gratifying way to stretch your capabilities and really be motivated to succeed.

Motivation here is defined as what will keep you moving day-to-day—the psychological characteristic that excites and causes you to act on something—in fact, it's the reason you act. So the idea is to a pick goal you'll *want* to aspire to, something that will keep you going with some degree of enthusiasm each day, so you can stay the course. No matter what you pick, your goal must stand the test of time. So get creative, add some interesting components that keep you going. Instead of just doing that walk around the park, try hiking one day a week (or month) or join a group that treks into unique areas. Instead of serving up bland food made the same way all the time, sign up for a course in low-calorie cooking, invest in a good, creative, low-cal cookbook, or borrow a few from a library.

Motivation may be considered mysterious, but we do know that it comes a lot more easily when it is attached to something meaningful.

When you feel right about the effort, you will seek to make it better—and see how it makes *you* better.

Achievable

While your goals should get you excited, they also need to be balanced, realistic, and set within an appropriate timeframe. Use your self-knowledge to determine what is really doable for you. You can test how realistic a goal is by asking yourself the question: *"Is it under my control?"* Goals like: "I'll get in such great shape, I'll be asked to model on the cover of *Vogue*" or "I'm going to be in the next Olympics" are lofty, but they require other people to recognize you and take certain actions—actions that are not under your control. You might be in good enough shape to be on the cover of *Vogue* or have the skills and experience to be in the Olympics, but achieving those goals may still be beyond your control.

Another form of this would be to make someone else responsible for your weight control or for you to take charge of someone else's. Goals like, "I'm going to get my spouse to stop forcing me to eat poorly," or "I'm going to get my coworkers to start exercising during lunch so that I will do it also" just won't work. The problem is that other people, no matter how close the relationship, are not obliged to follow your direction. You have no control over what they do, and trying to control someone or something you can't only invites frustration and resentment. Similarly, "I want my spouse to start eating healthier foods," may be a goal you have the power to influence, perhaps by selecting healthier foods and preparing them in healthier ways, but it is not a goal that can be *achieved* by you, for him (or her).

You can, however, create more realistic goals for handling other people's behavior. You might, for example, say, "The next time my husband orders cake at a restaurant and tries to get me to split it with him, I will either order something healthy for myself or perhaps go for a walk outside until he finishes." Or, if you're concerned about unhealthy eating and physical activity behavior at your office, you might decide to exercise three days a week at lunchtime and organize a jogging club.

A study of goal performance published in the academic journal *Ergonomics* indicated that performance was best when the assigned goals were somewhat difficult and labeled "do your best." Interestingly, performance was reduced when the goals were very easy, but it also diminished significantly when the goals were very hard. You need to find your *Achievable Goal Equilibrium.*

Never Say Never

To be achievable a goal can *never* be absolute. Don't ever say "I'll never have a piece of chocolate cake (or an order of fries or a bagel) again." To do that would be to hold yourself to a level of perfection that is simply not attainable in any aspect of life—including weight loss. And keep in mind that once you decide a food is forbidden, it's likely that you'll want it even more. Remember these few words *not* to use: *always, must, ever, never.*

I know a weight-loss consultant/nutritionist who recommends giving up friends who do not help you focus on exercise and food control. To her, this is a doable goal. But is it really realistic? To me it sounds a bit extreme. Cut off those in your social network because they aren't interested in helping you lose weight? I don't think so—that is simply not an achievable goal.

Here's another example. You don't want to set a goal of losing fifty pounds and running a marathon in a month if you've never even tried on a pair of running shoes. Yes, these goals may excite or motivate you plenty, but you need to be aware that things don't always happen that way, or that fast.

Setting unrealistic goals will discourage and frustrate you, and, as a result, you'll be more likely to abandon your weight-loss plan altogether. An achievable goal might be something like: "I'm going to lose twenty pounds over the next ten months by walking in the morning, replacing soda with unsweetened iced tea, going to a gym once a week to do strength training, and moving more during the day."

Set goals you know in your heart you can, and truly want to achieve. You have to be honest about your own capabilities, understand the nuts and bolts of the goals you set, and fit all the details into a manageable timeframe. And, if the amount of weight you have or want to lose is substantial, you need to be aware that it isn't going to happen in days or even weeks.

Don't Give In to Ego Threats

We all know how it feels to have someone threaten our ego, even in seemingly innocuous ways. If you've ever played golf or another sport with friends, you know what it's like to step up to the tee and hear someone say, "You'll never reach that green in one shot." Comments like that, generally used to psych out an opponent in sports, get your adrenaline pumping, your hands sweating, and affect your game. You may blast the ball to kingdom come to prove your friend wrong, and end up blowing it, overshooting it, or watching your perfect shot drop like a stone into the lake. Instead of hitting the best shot you can, you aim for the best shot in history, and thereby do worse than you would have had you stuck to your game plan. If you substitute your goal for the hole-in-one, you can see that such a response is self-sabotaging— a misdirected surrender to an ego threat.

Even people with high self-esteem are susceptible to what psychologists call "ego threats"—what you're apt to suffer when people you care about voice doubts about you or your abilities. Ego threats come from a variety of sources, but the most powerful come from the people closest to you, which is why they're so dangerous. You trust these people, and their undermining comments hurt you. Parents are infamous for posing ego threats: "You'll never be able to lose weight, so why try," or the seemingly less brutal, "You look good the way you are—don't bother losing weight." As a response to these threats, you might tell yourself, "I'm going to starve myself and lose seventy-five pounds in two months, if it's the last thing I do," or "I'm going to get my body looking like a supermodel." You can set unreasonably high standards for yourself and lose touch not only with what's important, but also with what's realistic when you're determined to prove someone wrong.

Or you can use ego threats as an excuse to give up. It's not unusual for people to internalize other people's doubts, thus jeopardizing their chances of achieving their goal. To do that, however, is to allow what other people think of your goals to be more important than what you think of yourself.

Sometimes the desire to prove doubters wrong may provide you with the energy you need to succeed just to prove to yourself you have what it takes. But you can't let other people's doubts or threats to your ego influence you in changing your goal in a way that would be detrimental to your achieving it.

How do you know if a goal is achievable? It's not always easy to identify goals that are balanced—neither too grand nor too small. When you set your goals, revisit some of the exercises you completed in Step 4. Look for diet and exercise patterns of behavior that actually worked for you in the past, as well as those that didn't work. If you want to determine what a realistic timeframe might be and/or which lifestyle adjustments you are really willing to make, you will have to ask yourself some questions.

How much weight can I lose each week and still remain in my comfort zone? An important factor in determining which goals are achievable is to recognize the skills you actually have. So, ask yourself, "What are my weight loss or exercise skills?" If you're not sure, try the simple exercise below.

What Are My Skills?

You can identify your skills by listing and analyzing five accomplishments that would be most helpful to your weight control. These might be anything related to physical activity, cooking, journaling, or organizing support groups, to name just a few. Be as specific as possible when preparing this list—don't just state an end result, but try to come up with the skill itself and how it will help you losing weight. For instance, you shouldn't simply state that you cooked a great roast chicken, that only tells me about a one-time event. It would be more helpful if you said, "I'm an excellent cook and make a great roast chicken, so that's one really healthy meal I can make at least once a week for myself and my family."

For each success, list the factors that motivated or excited you to excel in this situation, and the specific role you played. Look at the skill(s) you used for each one of your achievements. Are there any that stand out? Now review and reflect, and try to figure out how best to use these five skills to help control your weight.

Here are a few examples:

Cooking: I'm an excellent cook, and could buy some low-calorie cookbooks or even take a low-calorie cooking class that's offered at the local Y. It will be fun to try out new recipes, and my family loves to sample anything I make. This can help all of us eat healthier foods.

Tennis: I used to be a great tennis player; I really loved the sport and miss playing it. I could use the local high school courts or I could join an indoor court with the discount they give to employees of my company. I used to play every day when I was in college—I bet I could play two or three times per week. How about Saturday and Sunday, and one time during the week? I could even join a league. Let's see, if I played just twice a week for an hour per session, I'd be burning almost 1,000 extra calories each week. Not bad!

Journaling: I love to write, and journaling every day would be easy for me, I can keep track of everything I eat, all of my exercise, and my emotions. Then I could easily tally everything up and look for trends.

Group Support: Organizing groups is my thing. I was able to get my entire church to work on a clothing drive, and I organized a sub-group of the PTA to hold weekly meetings with the principal of my son's high school. I enjoy working with groups. Perhaps I could organize a weight-support group. That would be very helpful to me, having someone to talk to on a regular basis about my weight issues.

Which *five* skills can you apply to weight loss in your life?
1 . . . 2 . . . 3 . . . 4 . . . 5 . . .

Rewarding

Rewarding goals take into account the reasons for doing what you're doing. I call it understanding the Why. Why do you want to lose weight in the first place? I realize that might sound obvious, but trust me—many times it's not. I've found that people often convince themselves they're losing weight for one reason, when clearly it's about something else.

I was giving a lecture about goal planning when, at the end, one gentleman stood up and asked how he could quit smoking—quite a question. My first response was to ask him, "*Why* do you want to quit?" He looked at me as if I were a fool, and said, "Isn't it obvious? My health." He appeared to be in his early thirties, and since as a general rule I have found that most people under the age of forty are less concerned about their health than those over forty, I took a stab. "Okay, but are there any *other* reasons?"

Well, it turned out that he was the father of two-year-old twins. He went on and on about his boys having a greater chance of becoming smokers if a parent smoked, their dealing with the consequences of secondhand smoke, and the house smelling from cigarettes. Everyone in the room—except him—could see that his *real* reason for quitting smoking wasn't to improve his own health, but to improve the lives of his children.

Because he thought his reward for quitting would be his own improved health, every time he had to make a "micro" choice about whether or not to light up, his decision was simple. On the one hand he had cigarettes, with the benefits of relaxation, weight control, stimulation, and so on. On the other hand, there was the issue of his health—an intangible future reward that could be easily dismissed by a man in his thirties. What I did was to help him connect his reward for not smoking to the health and welfare of his twins. He may not have quit instantly, but his choice was a lot clearer. And with that clarification of the true reward he would get for quitting, the twins had at least a fighting chance. Having his rewards confused had been making it harder for him to break a negative pattern. And, like that father, to attain your goals you need to be clear about why you want to lose and control your weight, or why you want to exercise every morning. Having tangible, rewarding goals makes the process meaningful and helps you to stay on track.

To use the travel metaphor again, if you are on a road trip and all of a sudden you hit bad weather, or you get a flat tire, or anything negative occurs, one of the first things you might do is question the reason *why* you are even going on the trip. Remembering the reward—the beautiful hotel you'll be staying at or the lovely scenery you'll eventually get to enjoy—will help to keep you moving forward.

In the next Step, I'll provide you with an exercise called developing your "Life Preservers" that will help you to further define and identify your reason(s) *why*. You need to think about what it will be like to actually lose weight. How will you feel? What will you look like? Thinking about and understanding your rewards (the "Why") helps to establish an *emotional connection* to your goals that will help you get through the rough times, when you can easily be derailed.

Tactical

Reaching a weight-loss goal—or any goal—should never be about chance. Your ideal weight will not coincidentally materialize if you dream about it long and hard enough. Instead, you must want to lose the weight and maintain it badly enough to put a committed effort into making it happen. If a person is serious about achieving a goal, he or she needs to recognize that it requires techniques and tactics—again, not willpower or simply winging it.

Tactics are fundamental to the mechanics of reaching a goal. You need effort, persistence, and direction to prevail, and one will not work without the others. *Effort* is simply trying your best or making a serious attempt to move toward your goals. *Persistence* is staying the course even when the going gets tough. And finally, *direction* is the course you set to reach your objective. Effort without persistence is too short-lived, and effort without direction is merely activity or busywork. Persistence without direction will get you stuck in a rut leading nowhere in particular. And direction alone, without persistently putting forth an effort, dooms you to live, linger, and get stuck in the domain of dreams.

Tactics involve setting a plan of action that attempts to take all of the variables into account—removing the guess work. A tactical approach to problem-solving involves creative innovation rather than rote response.

Write It Down

One tactic for success is to give your ideas and goals words and an image to hold on to. To help you do that, try writing them down. Writing down your goals shows that you're truly committed to them; that they are real and important. Writing down your goals is the first step to making them happen. Keep in mind, you might find it uncomfortable writing your goals down for the very reason you *should* be writing them down—the fear of your goals becoming clearer. *That's why it's important for you to keep a notebook of all the exercises you've completed and notes you've taken from the pages in this book.*

Evaluated

Goals should be quantifiable and measurable in some way, meaning you should know if you're on the road to success, and when you're going to arrive. The more specific your goals are, the easier it is to evaluate your progress and determine if you're on track. For example, weighing yourself once a week will let you see at a glance if you're heading in the right direction. And keeping a food diary would be another good way to keep track of your energy balance (calories consumed versus calories burned.)

The National Weight Loss Registry has determined that almost all successful weight-loss maintainers have some kind of "five-pound warning system," a way of measuring and/or monitoring their weight before it is out of control. It could be something as simple as keeping a "thin" pair of pants or a dress rather than getting on the scale, but they all have some way of knowing if they are "slipping" and a backup plan they can put into action as soon as they receive their "fair warning."

When you're evaluating your progress, however, you need to be sure your methods are objective and accurate. Weighing yourself, for example, can be something of a double-edged sword. It helps to get on the scale once a week, but climbing on every day gives an inaccurate reading of your weight-loss progress because there are hour-to-hour variations in body weight. And reading the feedback recorded in your food diary can also be subject to inaccurate interpretation. You might be expecting too much too soon and judge the true state of your progress too quickly. Monitoring your weight-loss progress can be a lot like monitoring the return on an investment in the stock market. While it's important to look at yearly returns, checking on your investment every day could be less realistic than taking the longer view.

Reasonably spaced quantitative feedback lets you know where you stand in relation to a goal—whether you need to redouble your efforts, or whether it would be a good idea to come up with a whole new game plan.

And, when you're evaluating your progress, you should assess and reflect on your emotions as well, examining how you feel about the changes you're making in your life. Self-assessment and reflection are an important part of evaluation.

One Key to Smart Evaluations:
Asking the Right Questions

Questions are the most powerful tool when you're attempting to reflect and assess your progress. A good question should *not* be easy to answer. It should make you stop for a minute. It should set you off on a small journey into your mind. It's best if this journey takes you on unfamiliar paths. In that way, it opens up a potentially new way of thinking and seeing things. When you think in new ways, you grow better at thinking. The mind is a kind of muscle, and the more you use it, the stronger and more agile it becomes.

The questioning process is the cornerstone of inquiry. It helps to:

▶ Extend thinking skills
▶ Clarify understanding
▶ Gain feedback to learn
▶ Provide revision strategies
▶ Create links between ideas
▶ Enhance curiosity
▶ Motivate you to challenge yourself

Here are some questions to ask yourself as you begin the process of reflection. Be very specific in your answers.

1. Are these the permanent changes I am willing to make in my life to achieve my weight-loss goals?

2. What would I like to do that I am not currently doing to help me reach each of my goals?

3. What additional risks or challenges am I willing to take to achieve my goal of being a slimmer, newer me?

4. What is standing in the way of my making the changes I need to reach or maintain the body I want?

Now Analyze Your Answers:

Be ready to discuss your negative patterns without being defensive. Some people do their best reflecting out loud, talking with one other person or in small groups. Too large a group, however, tends to dilute the focus of whatever is troubling you and can invite the temptation to compare your life with others. Searching for similarities with others is totally beside the point. If you need to talk things out, my suggestion is that you do it one-on-one. Depending on your relationship with family members, you may turn to your parents, your spouse, or a sibling. Or you might be more comfortable talking with a good friend. You can learn a lot about yourself and generate new ideas by articulating a problem to another person.

Writing down your reflections and insights is a powerful tool. The action of writing transforms the reflection from a daydream to a concrete activity that can become the basis for decision making.

In addition to engaging in self-assessment and reflection, it's important to get feedback from other people because no matter how carefully you've planned, you may have overlooked some important aspect of reaching your goal. You can also lose perspective, which means you won't be an accurate judge of the quality of your own efforts. To regain that perspective, it can be useful to go to a few wise and thoughtful friends and advisers. Talking to others also prevents you from becoming bored and relieves some of the loneliness inherent in the pursuit of a goal.

One study found that schoolchildren preferred computer games that offered a clear goal and feedback about performance, and the same principle also applies to sports, in which score-keeping lets the players know where they stand.

But keep in mind that feedback should never become an excuse for not meeting your goals. If you acquire inaccurate feedback, it can be a substantial demotivator. Start-up businesses often convene a board of advisers who are experts in the field. You can do the same in the business of life—that is, assemble your own "board." Choose people who can aid and guide you appropriately. Your "board" should be genuinely concerned about your well-being, and if possible, one or two board members should demonstrate knowledge in your area of interest. If your goal is to lose weight, seek the advice of others you admire who have lost weight. If two or more people whose opinions you respect tell you you're way off base, it would be worthwhile for you to hear them out and ask for their advice.

But here, too, you have to seek a balance. At certain times, you just need to put your head down, charge forward, and go it alone without outside interference or help. If you've done your planning properly, you'll have faith in your own expertise.

The Goal of Self-Reflection

In his studies of extraordinary minds and extraordinary people, Howard Gardner, professor of education at Harvard, pioneered the notion of multiple intelligences. He wrote in his book *Extraordinary Minds*, "Extraordinary individuals stand out in the extent to which they reflect—often explicitly—on the events in their lives, large as well as small." Gardner said that an essential, common feature in great achievers throughout history is their ability and habit to think deeply about themselves, not in a selfish and narcissistic way, but in a way that brings them greater understanding of the human experience in general. Such people do not live their lives on automatic pilot, but instead, tend to bring a quality of thought and awareness to even their smallest deeds and actions, parts of life that many of us take for granted or overlook.

Revisable

After you evaluate and monitor/measure the goals you have set, you will want to revise those that don't make you *smarter*. Goals also need to be updated as circumstances change. For example, if you take on a new position that involves extensive travel, well, your goal to cook most meals at home will no longer be achievable and will need to be revised. You could get pregnant, divorced, married, promoted, demoted, suffer an injury—any number of circumstances could require revising your goals. And, in any case, you should formally review and revise your goals as necessary at least once a month, although you needn't wait until that time to make adjustments.

That said, it's also important to understand and recognize the difference between getting used to something new and the need to revise your goals. Trying something new may be uncomfortable at first, but if what you're doing allows you to remain within your comfort zone, it will become easier over time. If, on the other hand, it requires that you totally change who you are, it might never seem natural or comfortable for you. Making any type of change does involve adjustment. I hate to use a clichéd example, but it's just like buying a new pair of shoes. You know the story. At first you're excited, so you might grin and bear the pain of breaking them in. If they're a good fit, you'll get through it and wear them time and again. But if they're too big or too small or just plain too uncomfortable, after a while you'll begin to question whether or not they're worth the pain and trouble. The main point is that sometimes your goals need revising because they weren't the right goals to begin with and sometimes they need revising because circumstances have changed. Therefore, you need to make sure that your goals are well planned, using all the strategies I've provided.

Making Your SMARTER Goals a Reality

Goals can be tricky business. You don't want to err too far on the side of being unrealistic. But, on the other hand, you don't want to err by setting your sights too low, thereby spending a lifetime underachieving, only to end up wondering "what if" you had really applied yourself. Your goals, thankfully, are in your hands and not a matter of chance. So dare to take a proactive role in creating the world that lives in your dreams. It will not be handed to you.

All your goals should follow the guidelines above, but you still need different types of goals. Your goals should be broken down into micro, short-, mid-, and long-term, and *only you* can determine which is which. As a rule of thumb:

▶ Short-term goals: achieved in 1 month to 6 months

▶ Mid-term goals: achieved in 6 months to 2 years

▶ Long-term goals: achieved in 2 to 5 years.

Overall and Long-Term Goals

Setting your overall, long-term goal is the first decision you need to make. This would be the equivalent of picking a location for your next vacation; in order to start the planning process it helps to know where you're going.

You and I are planning your journey toward a life you can really live. But what does that look like? It's time to ask yourself, where are you going? And how will you get there?

Micro, Short-, and Mid-Term Goals

Micro goals are those little decisions of the moment that help to change your life. They're about deciding that the next time you go to the fridge you will reach for the mustard instead of the mayonnaise.

Short- and mid-term goals are those that get you to your long-term objective, the ones you have along the way. They should be created to keep you excited, motivated, and on-target, and to provide achievable objectives that bring you closer to your long-term goal.

You should start feeling good about your decision to lose weight right from the beginning. To help you do that, start each week by choosing a small goal you can meet within the next seven, ten, or fourteen days. You might aim to eat out one time next week at a restaurant featuring delicious, low-cal fish dishes. Your goal might be to not eat out more than twice a week. Or maybe you want to try a new cardio-sculpt class at the gym.

If you plan to push yourself hard some weeks, be sure to balance your program with other weeks of attainable short-term goals. Keep in mind that your short-term goals are stepping-stones to achieving your long-term goals.

It's also important to break your short- and mid-term goals down into categories that will help you to differentiate the various aspects of your larger, long-term goal. Weight control involves a variety of issues, including food choices, behavioral and psychological choices, and physical activity. Do you need all of these to come together to lose weight? Not necessarily, but the more of them you can control, the better your chances of success. Take a look at each of these categories below, so you have a starting point when you set your goals.

I. Food Choices

Think about how eating habits may be preventing you from losing weight. With this in mind, set one or two food goals that you would like to work on each week.

For example you might decide:

▸ I will not skip meals this week

▸ I will not snack on candy in the afternoon. Instead, I will have a fruit or a low-calorie bowl of cereal

▸ I will have wine with dinner only three nights this week, and I will keep it to one glass.

II. Behavioral and Psychological Issues

What is it about your lifestyle—or the way you think about yourself, food, or exercise—that is a barrier to weight loss? With this in mind, set one or two behavioral/psychological goals that you would like to work on each week.

Some examples of behavioral/psychological goals might be:

▸ I will only eat at the kitchen table when I'm at home. When I am tempted to eat in other areas of my home, I will remind myself of my long-term goals to lose weight and feel better about myself (Eating in just one or two places helps narrow down the number of spots in your home that you associate with food and eating.)

▶ I will not watch TV while eating (Eating consciously [not doing anything else while you eat] allows you to focus on what you're eating—actually enjoy it—and keep track of how much you're eating.)

III. Physical Activity

Developing physical-activity goals is imperative for any effective weight loss and weight-control program (and notice that I said *physical activity*, not exercise). These goals should be very specific in terms of how long, how much, and how hard you exert yourself. They need to be realistic and they should correspond to your overall goal. For example, if your objective is to lose thirty pounds in a year, and you're cutting about 200 calories a day on average from your diet, you might want to make up the deficit (about 90 calories), by doing an additional twenty minutes of walking each day, or taking the stairs instead of the elevator, or park in the farthest spot and walk to the entrance of the shopping mall, or walk three times a week. All these opportunities to move your body can help to make up the caloric deficit that will allow you to reach your goal.

Some examples of activity goals are:

▶ I will go walking for fifteen minutes during my lunch break at least three times this week

▶ I will walk up the three flights of stairs to my office every morning

▶ I will ride a bike with my daughter on Saturday and Sunday mornings

▶ I will run a 5K race one year from today.

Goals and Risk

Reaching your goals is not about gambling—unless, that is, your goal is to win a million dollars in the slot machines in Las Vegas. It's not a matter of random chance, no matter how hard you blow on the dice and pray. Reaching your goals requires using the techniques that will maximize your chances of achieving the weight loss you desire. It's a matter of getting SMARTER.

I'm not going to sugarcoat the message: *It's both brave and risky to have a goal.* To have a goal is to admit that you want something; and to yearn for something implies vulnerability, which is not necessarily a bad thing. It opens you up to the possibility of disappointment, failure, and rejection, which you might be inclined to fear. But having a goal is also taking a giant step toward being responsible. At first glance, being responsible can seem like a burden because it creates awareness—meaning that you emotionally and intellectually connect with the idea that *you* have the power to choose whether or not you lose weight. Eventually, however, you will come to understand that awareness leads to freedom—the freedom that goes along with increasing the likelihood of achieving your goal.

Think—and Make It Happen

"If one advances confidently in the direction of his dreams, and endeavors to live a life which he has imagined, he will meet with success unexpected in common hours." —Henry David Thoreau

"You are today where your thoughts have brought you, you will be tomorrow where your thoughts take you." —Ralph Waldo Emerson

I know it may be difficult for you to believe you can think your way to being fit. If it were only that easy, you're probably thinking, we'd all have daydreamed ourselves into new bodies by now. But the idea of using your reasoning mind *and* your imagination to control weight is not as far-fetched as you might think. In fact, an article in the *American Psychologist* has reported that "Mental stimulation provides a window on the future by enabling people to envision possibilities and develop plans for bringing those possibilities about."

In fact, athletes, business leaders, and other successful individuals all use visualization and mental rehearsal as well as self-talk—three methods for envisioning possibilities—to achieve performance goals, and these same tools will help you to reach your desired weight.

Visualization and Mental Rehearsal allow you to:

1. Define and develop your long term or overall goal by helping you to see it clearly
2. See an appealing image of an attainable future in your mind's eye, which will inform and inspire you to action
3. Fill in the details of what you need to do to reach those overall goals
4. Develop your Excuse Busters and other strategies to overcome obstacles that might stand in the way of reaching your weight-loss dream
5. Get through those micro choices, such as whether you should

wolf down that extra piece of cheesecake sitting on the table or pass it by

6. Anticipate how you're going to handle the rough times, such as Diet Busters, Eating Alarm Times, and Unconscious Eating by using a process known as Mental Rehearsal.

Visualization is a way for you literally to use your imagination to help you lose weight. The idea is to create an imagined, meaningful, detailed vision of your life *after* you've reached your goal weight. Like making a movie, you can create several vignettes, capturing a specific moment in time. If your goal is a trimmer you, imagine your body looking the way you want it to be in the future. This positive mental picture will help you keep the faith in the midst of the some of the tough food choices you'll be making.

Just be sure that your visualizations are not viewed through rose-tinted glasses. What you don't want to do is to idealize yourself beyond all possibility, which would mean that you've created an unrealistic overall goal.

Mental Rehearsal is a variation of visualization that allows you to *mentally practice* how you will behave when faced with difficult, weight-loss situations. It helps you make choices that support your weight-control efforts. If visualization gives you a picture of what you're shooting for, Mental Rehearsal prepares you to act in situations that might steer you in the wrong direction.

Let's go a little deeper with both strategies.

Daydreaming with a Purpose

Visualization is a tool that many people mock—until it works for them. They seem to believe that it's nothing more than daydreaming and, therefore, believe it's the mental equivalent of empty calories: not worth the time. Children, however, provide terrific examples of how to go about visualizing with gusto. When they talk about what they want to be when they grow up, they dive headlong into their fantasy worlds. They talk animatedly about their dream, and if they're old enough, they read about people who are prime examples of where they want to go. Kids can dress up or use toys to simulate the trappings of their chosen profession and easily transport themselves, figuratively, into that role. Well, you can do the same! The richness of the image and the sense that it can be real might not come naturally at first, but it's important to allow yourself this childlike gift. Don't worry—you still have it!

Film directors have been using this process since the birth of the movie-making industry. They call it "storyboarding," the process of illustrating every single shot in the entire film, detailing exactly how it will be filmed, the actors' expressions, and many other specifics that lead to the outcome they imagine.

Perhaps you have learned to censor your imagination, thinking you should not be squandering valuable time on mere daydreams. But this is *daydreaming with a purpose.* You are exploring who you are and getting to know your aspirations and desires. And, by the way, daydreaming *without* a purpose—taking note of what you think and fantasize—is not so bad either. It also provides you with information about yourself.

Albert Einstein wrote that, "Imagination is more important than knowledge," and told the story of how he used thought experimentation to visualize what the world would look like if one traveled at the speed of light. These imaginative leaps eventually led to his theory of spatial relativity. Of course, there was much hard work, perseverance, and many steps in between. But the journey might not have been possible without that first step.

Michelangelo also used a kind of visualization, which he called *intelleto.* The great artist believed that the form he sought in a block of marble already existed in the stone, and that he was just the means for allowing the true form of the stone to emerge. To see that true or ideal form, he needed *intelleto*—the capacity to see things as they truly are or are meant to be, which is also a kind of imagination. Imagination, not hard-nosed realism, is the starting point for many great achievements.

Athletes, too, are master practitioners of visualization. They have to be to succeed. As reported by Dan Levy in *USA Today,* world record–setting decathlete Dan O'Brien was the heavy favorite to win the gold medal at the 1992 Olympics in Seoul. He was on his way to the gold when the inconceivable happened—he failed to qualify in the pole vault. Since he was so far ahead in the other events, he was allowed to compete in the pole-vault competition as well, but he failed to clear the bar on all three attempts. He would have to wait four years before trying for the gold again in Atlanta in 1996. O'Brien rejected the idea of consulting a sports psychologist, but he worked on himself mentally during those years while continuing his physical training. "Milt Campbell, the 1956 gold medalist and the first black man to win a decathlon, told me that it takes place in your mind first," said O'Brien in an interview in the months leading up to the 1996 games. "If I don't wake up every day thinking I'm going to win the Olympic gold medal, I won't." When Dan O'Brien captured gold in Atlanta, he had already envisioned his victory many times.

Megan Quann, the sixteen-year-old who upset the defending Olympic champion, Penny Heyns of South Africa, in the one-hundred-meter breaststroke in Sydney is another example of an athlete's visualizing her victory. Quann had promised at the American Olympic trials that Heyns was "going down," and, every night before the event, she took a stopwatch to bed and visualized her race stroke by stroke. "I can see the tiles at the bottom of the pool, I can hear the crowd cheering, I can taste the water," Quann said of her ritual.

With visualization, you become the author of your future by actually designing what you want it to look like. One of the most effective ways to keep the faith in the midst of hard work is to hone your skills at:

▸ knowing how to achieve your desired outcome

▸ visualizing it's happening

▸ learning to use visualization as an asset when the going gets rough. During these difficult times, this mental view of the future is crucial.

As you anticipate your journey toward stress-free weight loss, having a clear mental image of what you want and expect of yourself—be it wearing a size 8 dress, developing a cut, muscular physique, or simply increasing your fitness and energy level—will help you to remember why you started on this process in the first place. And why is that so crucial to your success down the line?

Let's revisit that road trip we talked about in Step 8. If, for example, your mother called to tell you that you'd been invited to your second cousin's wedding in someplace you never heard of, that trip could make you a bit apprehensive—your destination is an unknown quantity and also very far from home. But then let's say someone who'd been there showed you photos of the place and it looked really beautiful and inviting. Maybe you also looked on the Internet and saw pictures of the boutique hotel where you'd be staying, with a fabulous pool, luxurious rooms, and an elegant lobby area.

As you viewed these images, the distance, and the trip, probably wouldn't seem so intimidating or burdensome any more, and your destination would no longer be completely unknown. You'd still never have been there, but you'd have made it more real by filling in the details and allowing yourself to imagine what it would be like once you'd arrived.

Now think of managing your weight the same way. You are about to go on a journey. Even though you might have dieted before, you've most likely never reached your actual destination (or else you wouldn't be reading this book!). So you need to think about what it feels like to reach that point. It's also important to think about the details, the obstacles, the stops along the way, and whatever else might influence your road trip toward a healthier body. Once you've mapped it all out and know what's in store for you, you'll be more prepared to progress. And the details you've imagined will help you to stay on course when you hit rough spots along your course to diet freedom.

Let me tell you a story about how visualization helped me. As you already know, for a long time I struggled with the fact that I wanted to be in better physical shape. One of the key issues I had to deal with was actually believing that I *could* ever be in the shape I wanted. I could dream about it, but I could never conjure up an image of what I would look like. No matter how hard I tried, I just couldn't make it clear in my mind. My possibilities were limited by the reality of what I saw in the mirror. I had no idea where I was going or what to aim for.

Then, finally, I broke through. I began to visualize myself in optimal physical shape and condition. It was more than just an image, I could actually see and understand how it would feel to be in the physical shape I'd always wanted to be in. It was the supreme "Aha!" moment because, not only could I perfectly envision a new, slimmed down, more attractive version of myself, I could also envision the path to that goal. From there, everything else fell into place because the benefits were completely apparent to me. The rewards were no longer vague and empty phrases, such as "I want to look better" or "feel more attractive." Visual imagery made the benefits tangible to me, and motivation ceased to be a problem. From then on, whenever I was discouraged or lost enthusiasm, I remembered the thoughts and feelings I'd collected from my visualization of achieving my goals.

I also used Mental Rehearsal to create a plan of action. I actually thought through how I was going to exercise each day, how I would prepare and cook my foods, and what I was going to do when I had an insatiable craving. I tried to go through every detail of what things would be like so that I would be prepared. I rehearsed what I was going to say at restaurants or to friends when they asked me about my "strange" or "new" eating habits.

One way to keep the faith when the going gets tough is to hone your skills at visualizing the outcome—and to *keep that vision close at hand*. When you can see an appealing image of an attainable future, it informs and inspires your actions, and helps to coordinate your plan and goals. But that is not to say you should—or even can—live entirely in what may seem at first to be the very distant future.

Creating the Details for Short- and Mid-Term Goals

While you're visualizing what it will be like when you reach your long-term goal, you also need to be filling in the details by visualizing your short- and mid-term goals. For instance, if your overall goal is to lose fifty pounds, you need to be very specific about how you will do that, meaning you need to include time frames, what types of foods you're going to eat, the types of food you're going to cut out, any physical activity you may add—in other words, all the details. While you're mapping all of this out, you are, in effect, *visualizing*. Use visualization techniques to help fill in *all* the details for short- or mid-range goals.

Creating Your Own Life Preservers

There will be times when you have to make an immediate decision in a tough and tempting situation, times when even your best-laid plans simply won't cut it and life, such as it is, will threaten to take you off track. Those are the times when having a well rehearsed, clearly defined mental image of the future can prove to be a real Life Preserver. Because it's already in the back of your mind, making the decision to stay on track will be automatic.

A Life Preserver is a *positive,* visualized, and fully imagined future event, situation, or circumstance that is tough enough to stand up to your worst food crisis. With your Life Preservers in tow, you'll have the empowerment you need to emotionally and mentally walk away from the fudge, the fries, or the fettuccini.

Creating a Life Preserver helps you in those make or break moments to remember why you wanted to lose weight in the first place as well as to remain focused on your goal.

In an interview in *Men's Fitness*, Ken Ross, a former fitness coach for the U.S. Olympic team, talked about using visualization: "Imagine it's one year from today, and everything has gone according to plan . . . Ask yourself how your life would be different," Ross advises. "How would it feel to look in the mirror? How would you feel buying clothes for your new body? . . . Imagining a successful future creates passion," Ross says.

This snapshot from your future life will help you to focus on your overall goal. And seeing the results helps to fill in the details of how you'll get there.

I'm going to ask you to develop three vignettes or visualizations of something that could happen in your future once you achieve your goal. The purpose of these visualizations is to have three different motivational scenarios you can keep in your back pocket, purse, or wallet, to pull out when you're having a tough time sticking to your plan. These are the images you will cling to when you find yourself desperately in need of dieting salvation, so make them as compelling, inspiring, and clear as you possibly can. They will, after all, have some powerful forces to stand up to: your own double-chocolate fudge birthday cake, the cheese platter during cocktail hour at your friend's house, those tasty mayo-heavy side dishes your mother whips up for Sunday dinner, and every candy maker specializing in truffles sold by the box.

Make Them Foolproof

1. **Make them *detailed:*** You should be able to smell, see, and hear this future moment. What will you look like when you lose the weight? How will you feel? How will your life be different?

2. **Make them *compelling:*** If these visualizations are compelling and inspiring, they'll really mean something to you when you're in

need. (Remember, your desire for the "bad" stuff is not going to go away anytime soon, so the more compelling the image, the better it will hold up against your "dreamiest" food desires.)

3. List *events*:   Use upcoming events as a way to set the stage for your visualization. For example, imagine seeing an old friend at a reunion after losing thirty pounds, or going to a doctor's appointment and hearing that your cholesterol and blood pressure have decreased, which means that you've significantly lowered your risk for cardiovascular disease as well as diabetes. Here's an example from a client who told me: "I ran into my ex-husband at the mall. I hadn't seen him in years, and he didn't even recognize me at first. Boy, did it feel great to be sixty pounds lighter and feeling wonderful!"

4. Write them down and keep them *available*:   Make sure your visualizations are at your fingertips at all times. Laminate the page or note card, use a page in your date book, or enter them in your PalmPilot or electronic organizer. *Keep them handy* so you can refer to your written list when you have a craving or are tempted to go overboard.

5. Relax: Don't worry if you can't visualize a slimmer, healthier you right away; experts say that it can take some time. Instead, start with the future event itself, and over time the rest of the details will work themselves out.

Here are a few examples to help you get started:

I've just come from an art opening. I'm wearing a size 8 turquoise sheath dress and carrying a matching vintage, beaded handbag. It's a summer night, and I pull up to the restaurant, pay the driver, and step out of the cab. My date is waiting for me by the door. I walk toward him with a confidence I haven't felt in years. I am fit and healthy and I know that no matter how this evening turns out, I will return home tonight feeling good about myself.

I'm pretty nervous, going to the doctor again—I just can't bear the thought of finding out that I have diabetes. Knowing that my mom had the disease, and knowing what it did to her . . . my gosh! I really am nervous . . . I even put my sweater on backward. I was going to have my husband drive me, but I

really thought it would be better just to go by myself. After six months of work-
ing out and changing my lifestyle I'm really feeling pretty confident, and los-
ing those thirty-six pounds helps, too. I really never thought I could do
it—work out and eat better—but it hasn't even been that difficult.

Wow, I'm here at the doctor's office already. I sit in the waiting room . . . I
always hated the waiting room . . . sitting and thinking about all the possible
diseases I could have. Finally, the nurse calls me into the examination room.
I've already had all the tests done, and this is the exam that'll give me the an-
swers! Then I hear the words from the doctor that make me cry: "Linda, you're
amazing! You managed to lower your cholesterol, your blood pressure is great,
your bone density is improved, and your sugar levels are fine! You really have
changed your life and you look wonderful." I really feel good about myself be-
cause I'd been worried about my health and what would happen to my kids if
I weren't around to take care of them.

My first husband used to make me feel terrible about my weight problem.
Bob was always telling me I could never lose weight because I was "weak" and
had no control over my life. He would tell me he was going to find himself a
new "hot" woman who didn't look like a "beached whale." Sometimes he'd say
it as a joke, but I knew he was serious, and he actually did end up leaving me
and marrying (and divorcing) a younger, thinner woman.

I haven't seen him in a few years. I've heard he was having a hard time af-
ter his latest divorce, but I'm past all that. I've changed my life—taken con-
trol. I've lost about fifty pounds, I'm exercising, and I've gone back to school.
Everything about my life is different, and I look great even if I do say so myself.
Well, one day I'm headed to the mall after a long day of running around. I en-
ter the mall by the food court—and that's when he sees me. He gasps, almost in
shock at how much weight I've lost—and how good I look . . .

Now you try it. Take out your notebook. Pick one Life Preserver, sit in
a comfortable environment, allow yourself to dream about it, then
write down all your thoughts—every last one of them. Continue to add
to the visualization, including more details and feelings, and incorporate all your senses until your Life Preserver takes on the quality of a
real experience.

To get started, ask yourself the following questions:

1. *What will I look like when I lose weight permanently?*
2. *How will I feel?* Think about how you felt when you accom-
    plished things in other areas of your life. Try to transfer those re-

warding feelings to having succeeded in reaching your weight-loss goal

3. *How will my life be different?* Think about specific things you do in your everyday life—showering, going to the supermarket, driving in a car, taking the bus, walking up a flight of stairs, etc. How will these be different in your new, improved body?

4. *How will others in my life react to me?* Be specific. Name names. Your spouse, children, parents, friends, the wait staff at restaurants you frequent. They all matter

5. *What will it be like to have a clean bill of health and feel better physically?* These benefits may seem somewhat intangible. Be as specific as possible. You can visualize having more energy, going to the doctor, and finding out that you are not a high-risk candidate for diabetes.

The end result should be three different Life Preservers. Each one should be a clear, polished, tangible experience in your mind.

Helpful Tools for Developing Your Life Preservers

As the Spanish expression goes, "Living well is the best revenge." Come on—dish the dirt! We all have someone from the past we want to look great for and then walk away from. Nobody said your Life Preserver had to be worthy of a good works medal or even polite, cocktail-party conversation. The purpose of this living-well visualization is for it to be clear, emotional, and *inspiring for you alone.* And as history (as well as any Charles Bronson movie) has shown, revenge can be an incredibly effective incentive.

So who is it that you'd like to run into in your Life Preserver visualization? An ex-boyfriend or girlfriend, your current or ex-spouse? An old friend who's done well and married the person you once loved? A former coworker who was a ferocious competitor and made trouble for you? Reward is the key here! Dig out the old photos. Do you have any pictures of yourself at your goal weight? Old photos are vivid reminders that, *yes!,* your body *is* capable of looking like that again! (However, remember to keep a realistic perspective when using old photos as a motivational tool. Losing weight is not necessarily going to make you look twenty years younger, but you *can* feel twenty years more confident!)

If you've never been at your goal weight during your adult life, it might be more difficult for you to imagine what you're working toward in terms of physical appearance. In that case, look through magazines to find a picture of someone who has features similar to yours, and who is at your ideal body weight. Use this photo as a tool for developing a clear vision of yourself at your future weight. (But please leave body-type extremes like Calista Flockhart or Arnold Schwarzenegger out of this exercise, even if your *face* is a similar shape or you have a tendency to build muscle. Remember, SMARTER goals are those that are *realistic*.)

Still Stuck? More Tips to Help Create Your Life Preservers

Having trouble dreaming up your Life Preservers? Try the following:

▸ Sit in a comfortable, quiet place.

▸ Close your eyes and let yourself dream. Your dreams may seem fuzzy or disjointed at first. Don't try to force them into any sort of coherent logic just yet. Let your thoughts drift wildly. See how far you can go.

▸ Concentrate on and imagine what you would like to do, accomplish, achieve—or simply just let yourself fantasize and your mind wander.

▸ If you're having trouble creating visualizations that would be valuable to you, or if you have a hard time imagining yourself carrying out your dreams, try the following:

— Use your imagination and all your senses to develop an image of your future self that you find truly motivating. Make the images of your daydream bigger, closer, more colorful. Add pleasant sounds, an encouraging voice, or whatever will make the visualization more attractive to you. Keep doing this until you are strongly attracted to this visualization and feel an emotional connection—until it's almost as clear in your mind as a fresh memory.

— Think about what it will be like to actually live the life you see in this visualization. Fill out some of the contours of your daydream. What does your future look and feel like? What would it be like to live in the world you are conjuring up for yourself? What kind of people will be there? How will they act? How will you interact with them? Give this a great deal of thought and detail, and include sounds, smells, feelings, and tastes. Make the image colorful, detailed, rich, and vibrant. In the end, the visualization in your mind's eye should be so clear that you will have no doubt about what you really want.

— Now, move beyond the external vision of yourself and put yourself inside this new you. What kind of clothes will you be able to wear as a result? Will looking fitter impact your career or social life? Think of how good it will feel to be in great shape.

— Let yourself lose control of the internal reels every once in while and see where they take you. Remember, you are the director of your movie. If you don't like where the story is going, you can rewind, recut, and revise the script.

— Write down some of the images. Which ones were the strongest? Which ones made you feel best?

— Stay on track. If negative or self-sabotaging thoughts come into your mind, replace them with the increasing feelings of success and competence you create as you take each step.

Revisit old memorabilia. Maybe you have a high school trophy, an achievement-award certificate, a yearbook photo, a pair of race-winning sneakers—anything that might remind you of a goal you once reached or a state of physical fitness you attained when you were younger. Summon up the feelings you had then, how the world looked to you, and how your body felt.

Set the stage. Maybe you already have the staging set for the visualization you're using as a Life Preserver, and your "new self" is the only missing piece. Perhaps you're working up to a trip to Hawaii and plan to spend the whole time there in an attention-getting bikini. Or your wedding is a few months away. Maybe there's a specific race you're training for. Well, it's time to gather up the airplane tickets, wedding invitations, and entry forms—and use them as reminders and tools for imagining yourself as an *active player*.

The stage can also be set with other upcoming events you're aiming to look good for. Reunions can be great motivators. Do you have a high school, college, or family reunion coming up? Be detailed: Imagine whom you'll run into and what you'll wear. But don't let this be your sole motivator. If you don't have other, more long-term motivations in mind, the buffet table at your goal event is likely to be your first stop on the road back to where you started!

Having an "Aha!" Moment

A study done at the University of Colorado Health Science Center and reported in the *American Journal of Clinical Nutrition* reports that the majority of weight-loss maintainers' success was preceded by a "trigger event or critical incident." These events varied from "medical (i.e., doctor told them to lose weight), emotional (i.e., someone made a derogatory comment about their weight), or a life event (i.e., a new baby)." A trigger event can be a humiliating personal disaster, such as a spouse leaving you. It can be something as casual as overhearing a hurtful comment about your girth at a shopping mall. Or it can be an invitation to a reunion that motivates you to get into the best shape to impress people who haven't seen you in a long time.

Whatever its origin, however, a trigger event is invariably an "Aha!" moment that causes you to examine your life from a new perspective so that you gain a new insight and see yourself as you really are. It's a higher level of perception. Suddenly, you are enlightened. You know that the course your life has been taking is no longer acceptable and that you need to change.

A trigger makes you reflect on where you've been and where you are going. My own "Aha!" moment was actually a string of uncomfortable events, including breaking up with a girlfriend, my father's being diagnosed with diabetes, moving, and assorted other goodies. It was reflection time. I was unhappy with where I was, not happy with where I'd been, and not very excited about the future. I was determined to avoid diabetes, a disease that runs in my family, to change my appearance, and to move my life to a new place.

But whatever it is, like mine and those listed above, a trigger event or "Aha!" moment generally springs from a *negative, rock-bottom* experience. For instance, maybe you gained forty pounds after having a baby and now that baby is ten years old and you've gained and lost that forty pounds about twenty times. Your doctor has just told you that if you don't lose the weight, you'll be a prime candidate for a heart attack. That pronouncement will, no doubt, trigger a significant amount of self-reflection. That's a catalyst or trigger. The "Aha!" moment comes when you realize *how to change the patterns that keep getting you into the same kind of yo-yo weight gains and losses.*

But you don't always have to hit rock bottom before you see the light. You can help to *manufacture* your own alternative triggers and "Aha!" moments by creating compelling Life Preservers for yourself, thereby creating something *positive* to help motivate you to shed the pounds. One of the beneficial side effects of visualization is that, by allowing you to actually see the light at the end of the tunnel, it can provide one of those moments when you know instantaneously, after years of following deeply ingrained patterns, not only that you *will* make a change, but also *how* you're going to do it.

Practice Makes Perfect—Roadblock Anticipation

If visualization gives you a picture of what to shoot for, Mental Rehearsal provides preparation for situations that might steer you in the wrong direction. Or, as Louis Pasteur said, "Chance favors the prepared mind."

Lights, camera, action! If your life were a movie, you'd be the star, the screenwriter, the director, and the location manager, among other roles. Unfortunately, however, when you're in an Unconscious or Mindless Eating situation, facing one of your Eating Alarm Times, or confronting a Diet Buster, it might seem as if the movie of your life were a remake of *Groundhog Day*. You wake up every morning and it's the same day over and over and over again—until, one day, you get it. Worse yet, it might feel as if you've been cast in the role of your own worst enemy!

If you feel that the weight-loss plot of the film of your life is more like a disaster flick than a comedy, it's up to you to give it a happy ending. And you can do that. One of the keys to maintaining your focus and sense of purpose during potentially disastrous moments is having determined in advance how you're going to react. And you can do that through the process of Mental Rehearsal.

Mental Rehearsal or Roadblock Anticipation allows you to practice responding to difficult weight-loss situations in a way that supports rather than undermines your lifestyle change. Mental rehearsal also shows you what it will feel like to be free of a particular overeating shackle—such as eating your way through an entire row of Oreo cookies to relieve the pressure of a bad day at work.

Mental Rehearsal "definitely enhances learning," says Jean Williams, a sports psychologist at the University of Arizona and former president of the American Association for the Advancement of Applied Sports Psychology. "You can learn new techniques faster than if you just do physical practice, and you can refine performance."

Most of the world's top athletes engage in Mental Rehearsal before a big event. Six-time Ironman triathlon winner Mark Allen, for example, goes on spiritual retreats as he prepares for the grueling event. He focuses on how he will overcome the pain, and trains himself to block it out. World-class skiers imagine each run down the slope, perfectly executing each turn, to train their bodies to do the same when they actually compete. And, according to the *American Journal of Surgery*, surgeons who practice their skills using Mental Rehearsal perform better in the operating room.

Everyone engages in some type of Mental Rehearsal throughout the day. When you imagine getting home and relaxing after a long, hard day, or when you think about how you're going to respond to your child's bad report card, these are, in a way, forms of Mental Rehearsal.

Mental Rehearsal can also reduce anxiety before and during a performance. Psychologist and former all-American swimmer, Marcia Middel, PhD, says she uses these techniques to help athletes and musicians overcome performance anxiety.

And, in his autobiography, *Second Wind: The Memoirs of an Opinionated Man*, basketball Hall-of-Famer Bill Russell, the only man to win a staggering eleven NBA championships, described an experience he had at age eighteen while watching a basketball game from the bench:

> Something happened that night that opened my eyes and chilled my spine. I was sitting on the bench watching Treu and McKelvey the way I always did. Every time one of them would make one of the moves I liked, I'd close my eyes just afterward and try to see the play in my mind . . . I'd try to create an instant replay on the inside of my eye-

lids . . . On this particular night, I was working on replays of many plays including McKelvey's way of taking an offensive rebound and moving to the hoop . . . Since I had an accurate vision of his technique in my head, I started playing with the image right there on the bench, running back the pictures several times and each time inserting a part of me for McKelvey.

Finally, when I saw myself making the whole move, I ran this over and over. When I went in the game, I grabbed an offensive rebound and put it in the basket just the way McKelvey did. It seemed natural, almost as if I were stepping into a film and following the signs.

How does it work? A study by Alvaro Pascual-Leone, MD, PhD, professor of neurology at Harvard University, demonstrated the process. He monitored the brain patterns of three groups of volunteers as they learned a simple five-finger exercise on the piano. One group practiced the exercise daily for two hours while the second group sat at the piano for two hours just hitting the keys without learning anything. Those in the first group showed tremendous changes in the part of the brain dealing with the use of hand muscles. The volunteers who just tickled the ivories aimlessly showed little or no change in their brain patterns.

But the biggest surprise came from volunteers in the third group. These people were taught the piano exercise, but were allowed to rehearse it only mentally, *not* manually, while looking at the keyboard. After five days, their brain patterns were identical to those of the volunteers who actually practiced the melody.

Mental rehearsal works because it actually gives your brain a chance to rehearse your life choices. It's a way of anticipating and preparing for future events you know are going to occur, and taking responsibility for how you will respond to them. What you're really doing here is thinking ahead. Can you prepare for every possible eventuality? I doubt it, but the more you plan, think about, and anticipate those rough times, the more you will stay in your weight-control zone.

Make no mistake, giving in to Unconscious or Mindless Eating, Eating Alarm Times, and Diet Busters is not just about a failure of willpower. Many of the choices you make come out of deeply rooted patterns of behavior. To overcome such ingrained behavior, you must train yourself to have new reflexes and reactions. In a way, it's like learning to ride a bicycle. When you learned to walk as a baby, you kept falling over until you developed an innate sense of balance that allowed you to remain upright without thinking about it. When you learn to ride a bike, you need to develop new ways of balancing in order not to fall off, so you keep on practicing until riding a bike seems as natural as walking. Luckily, however, you don't have to physically practice standing in the buffet line at your best friend's wedding in order to learn how to turn down fattening food. Instead, you can rehearse the scenario in your mind. Here's how Sharon, one of my clients, used Mental Rehearsal to prepare for a regular social engagement:

> My friend Laura and I normally meet at an Italian restaurant for lunch on Tuesdays and Thursdays. Their standard menu has too many tempting dishes I know I should avoid, so I'm going to phone the restaurant tomorrow morning before work and request a low-fat, low-calorie meal. I'll order fish or chicken grilled with no oil or butter, along with a salad. I'll tell them I'm embarrassed to ask the waiter in person, and to please have this meal ready for me every Tuesday and Thursday. I'll call ahead to make sure they prepare it for me on those two days.
>
> I imagine myself getting in the car to go to the restaurant. It's a sunny day, I'm in a good mood, and I'm determined to eat well at lunch. I put in my favorite CD and sing along as I drive. As I get to the parking lot I make sure I remind myself to eat well, because I know I'll feel better afterward and look better in the long run. I imagine myself walking up the stairs and sitting down with my friend. The bread plate comes, and I pass it by. Instead, I ask the waiter who always serves us to bring out a plate of cut-up vegetables, and I snack while we wait for our food. Plus, I ate an apple before I got in the car and drank a small bottle for water, so I wasn't starving anyway.
>
> Leaving the restaurant having eaten the healthy meal I'd requested and not going off my life program, I feel as if I'm on track. Let's see . . . now I'm in my car on my way back to the office. Instead of feeling bloated, guilty, and disappointed with myself, I feel accomplished, like I'm on my way to living a healthy life, losing weight, looking better . . . I even imagine myself fitting into a size ten.

When you imagine the script in advance, you'll be prepared to act and react as if it had already happened. By empowering yourself through Mental Rehearsal, you actually increase your mind's ability to make healthy choices when you're tempted to do the opposite. Plus, you also get a glimpse of how good you'll look—and feel—having successfully resisted temptation, which will help you to create new automatic behaviors.

Just Say "No!"

Being able to say "no" effectively is one of the most important skills you can have as you work to improve your eating and exercise habits because, the fact is, even the most well-meaning people won't always be as supportive as you'd like. Imagine, for example, that you're at the movies and your friend asks you to share a large popcorn. He or she might think doing that would make you happy—that it would be a treat. You have to ask yourself if that's really what *you* want, and, if it isn't, you have to be ready to say no.

To Mentally Rehearse just such a situation, write down three occasions when you were with friends, family, or loved ones who put you in a situation that made you uncomfortable about saying no to food.

Here's an example: *I was at a big family dinner and everyone was eating huge plates of food. My relatives kept nagging me to eat more, and when I declined they'd say things like "Oh, come on, it's a holiday and I know you love my cheesecake." When it comes to food, my relatives just won't take no for an answer.*

Now it's your turn:

1.

2.

3.

The key is to prepare responses to these types of situations so that you'll be armed with an automatic answer the next time one rolls around. By being prepared in advance, you'll have a better chance of controlling the outcome.

So write down your answers to the three situations you described above. I'll get you started with my own.

Situation: *My relatives want me to eat everything in sight, even when I tell them I'm not hungry.*

What I say: *I do love your cooking, but I'm really full and I couldn't eat another bite. No cheesecake for me!*

> What I'm thinking: *Sure, the cheesecake looks good, but the fact is, I'm not really hungry. And I really want to reach my weight-loss goal.*
> Now you do it:
>
> Situation:
> What you say:
> What you're thinking:

Remember Scott, who traveled for his job? Well, he came up with a real plan for helping himself to achieve his goals by using Mental Rehearsal. In addition to calling the hotels in advance to find healthy restaurants in the area, taking sandwiches onto the plane, and finding out if the hotel had a gym, he also Mentally Rehearsed eating his sandwich on the plane, walking into the restaurant and ordering healthier foods, and putting on his sneakers to work out in the exercise room.

Developing Your Own Mental Rehearsal

First of all, go back over the Unconscious or Mindless Eating, Eating Alarm Times, and Diet Busters you discovered when you were doing your detective work in Step 5. You're going to think of each one in turn, but this time you're going to mentally rehearse an ideal ending in which you make healthy-food choices, feel great, and stay in control of your thoughts, actions, and emotions.

Here is a step-by-step guide to Mental Rehearsal:

1. Choose one of your Unconscious or Mindless Eating behaviors, Eating Alarm Times, or Diet Busters and develop a rough sketch of how you'd like to change your behavior in that scenario—include the thoughts, emotions, and actions you want in your ideal version.

2. Now start to add in a few details. Break these details down into imaginary steps. Think how you would act and behave to move toward this very targeted goal, and write it down. Be specific and go into the nitty-gritty details. Don't spare a thought, no matter how insignificant it might seem.

3. Now you're ready to write a step-by-step description of exactly what your ideal experience would actually be like.

Be creative and thoughtful about the process. Sharon, for example, came up with an alternative to the bread plate. You must really understand the experience from beginning to end. Consciously visualize what it will take for you to get through this situation. When you think through the details, you give yourself time to plan in advance. Don't fly blind, but give yourself this advantage. You deserve it.

4. Once you have the general script down, go back to make the experience really come alive. Use all your senses. Becoming an expert in focused visualization and Mental Rehearsal requires you to look both inward and outward.

5. Revisit your Mental Rehearsal frequently. Give it positive energy with strong affirmations and feelings that the goal is real and reachable.

6. Rerun that scenario in your head whenever you find yourself about to live out the situation you've rehearsed. The details should be as familiar to you as the words and notes to your favorite song.

After you feel comfortable with the scenario you've developed for a particular situation, stop to congratulate yourself before going on to Mentally Rehearse the next one. You can even use this same technique as an Excuse Buster the next time you find yourself tempted to skip your morning walk or other planned physical activity by Mentally Rehearsing how good you'd feel after a workout.

What you're doing through Mental Rehearsal is creating new *automatic* responses to replace your previous patterns—the ones that had been keeping you fat. Just think about it logically. If you are used to getting the dessert menu at a restaurant and ordering dessert, you do it unconsciously because it's a pattern or habit. If you do nothing to intervene, you will continue to do the same thing over and over. Now, if you rehearse a different outcome—for instance, ordering cut-up fruit, coffee, or no dessert at all—you have created a *new* automatic response to the dessert menu. And if you're worried that your life will lack spontaneity as a result of all this planning and preparation—don't fret. In fact, you will always have choices; all you're doing is deciding in advance what that choice will be with regard to food and physical activity.

Above all, remember: If you fail to plan, you plan to fail. Rehearse and you'll get the gold!

Go to your notebook and write down *three* Mental Rehearsals for each one of your Diet Busters, Eating Alarm Times, and Unconscious Eating behaviors.

Diet Buster Mental Rehearsal

My Diet Buster is _____

My Mental Rehearsal is _____

Eating Alarm Time Mental Rehearsal

My Eating Alarm Time is _____

My Mental Rehearsal is _____

Unconscious Eating Mental Rehearsal

My Unconscious Eating occurs _____

My Mental Rehearsal is _____

Affirmation and Self-Talk

An affirmation is a strong, positive statement that assumes something desirable *is in fact true*. The act of using words and talking to yourself about yourself makes the situation more real than just visualizing it, however detailed the vision might be.

Whether you're aware of it or not, most people's lives are accompanied by a stream of internal commentary. An example would be constantly telling yourself, "I can't lose weight—it's just too difficult" or "I'll never be able to get out there and walk every day" or "I can't eat at a restaurant without pigging out on the bread basket."

Would you ever get on an airplane once you'd overheard the pilot say, "I don't think I can make it all the way to Florida. I just know I'm going to crash, I'm so scared." No, of course not. And aren't you the pilot of your own life? You're the one in charge. Do you really want to be the one convincing yourself that you won't succeed? Granted, there are times when it's natural to feel insecure about your undertakings—but don't be your own worst enemy.

A study in the *Journal of Sports Sciences* divided golfers of high and low skill into two groups. Both groups executed a series of putts. Those in the first group were asked to believe and tell themselves they would succeed, and those in the second group were instructed to think and tell themselves they would *not* succeed. The investigators found that the players they'd instructed to engage in negative self-talk performed much worse than those who used positive self-talk regardless of their skill level. If you're constantly putting yourself down and berating yourself with negative talk, try to:

▸ Make yourself aware of your own thoughts

▸ Replace negative thoughts with positive ones

▸ Reinforce those positive thoughts and feelings with affirmations.

When practiced and repeated over time, affirmations can alter your mental climate and empower you to make changes in your life. Most of you are familiar with the children's book *The Little Engine That Could*, in which a humanized choo-choo train is able to surmount challenges that seem impossible by chanting over and over, "I think I can, I think I can." This is a parable about the power of affirmations. And as automotive pioneer Henry Ford said in a similar vein, "If you think you can't, you're right."

A study at the University of Alberta, Edmonton, found that some active people "expressed as much negative self-talk as did inactive people. However, they differed in their ability to balance each issue with strong, positive thinking based on previous personal successes and direct experience of benefits." This is exactly why having Excuse Busters available is so important—you need to have the *answers* to that negative self-talk so that you can override it rather than letting it drag you down.

Jim Johnson, a sports psychologist for professional sports teams, teaches athletes to replace negative self-talk with positive statements. If you make a mistake, don't scold yourself, he suggests. "Acknowledge your frustration, let it go, and focus on the next play." He instructs the players to constantly reassure themselves with thoughts like, "I am a major league baseball player," or "I'm going to throw nine innings today." Like most sports psychologists, Johnson believes that baseball is only

25 percent physical. "The difference between Triple A ball players and big leaguers is mental," he told *U.S. News and World Report.*

You, too, can reap the benefits of reassuring self-talk. It will help you to deal with your frustrations and keep you on track. The key to using affirmations effectively is to overcome what I call "the corniness factor." You may be reminded of Al Franken's goofy and hilarious *Saturday Night Live* character Stuart Smalley, whose mantra was: "I'm good enough, I'm smart enough, and gosh darn it, people like me."

You may even laugh at yourself when you start to use affirmations, and that's okay. Affirmations do sound funny at first. Eventually, however, as you become more comfortable with the idea of yourself as someone who can achieve your dreams, you'll become more comfortable with the strategies to reach them. And at the very least, if you don't feel comfortable with proactive self-affirmations, make sure to put a stop to negative self-talk—telling yourself you can't do something.

When you begin to think of affirmations, you should write them down in the present tense and repeat them to yourself either as a kind of meditation or whenever you're experiencing a situation that normally upsets you, stresses you out, or damages your self-esteem. For the person who experiences problems on the job, such an affirmation might go something like: "I am a competent person who is capable of succeeding at this task." For an overweight person who struggles with a poor body image, the affirmation might be: "I am a beautiful person and I deserve to look the way I want to look." The repetition of such positive statements will eventually lead to a change in the way you view yourself and your own capabilities. Gradually, the mind responds affirmatively and you begin to experience your intended results.

Your Mind Is a Powerful Thing

Visualization, Mental Rehearsal, and Self-Talk are powerful mental strategies for changing physical circumstances. When you're making significant changes in your life by creating a livable diet and increasing your physical activity, you need all the help at your disposal. Use these, along with Excuse Busting and SMARTER goal-setting to empower you so that you can make the best use of the tools you were given in Part 1 and ensure that you stay off the diet roller-coaster for the rest of your life.

◄◄◄ STEP 10 ►►►

Create a Blueprint

"Choose the life that is most useful, and habit will make it the most agreeable."

—Francis Bacon

You've learned a lot. Not only do you now have new insights into your own "fat" patterns, but you have also acquired all the tools and strategies you need to break those patterns and create new, automatic ones that will keep you in the permanent-weight-loss club forever. Now it's time to organize that information (which you might already have done), put it all together, and create a comprehensive blueprint for implementing and achieving your goals.

To help you do that, I've put together a sample organizational chart you can use as a template for filling in the steps you will take to reach success.

The Overall Goal

Lose thirty-five pounds forever!

Mid-Term Goal

Lose twenty pounds in the next six months and change my style of eating and activity.

The Strategy, Specific Details, and Subgoals

Twenty pounds in six months is a 70,000 calorie deficit, which translates to about 250 calories per day. So, if my substitutions add up to about 200 calories per day (e.g., one less medium fast-food soda), and I increase my physical activity by about fifty calories per day (e.g., walking for an additional ten minutes), I'm set.

Results of Three-Day Food Challenge, Possible Foods I Can Substitute

An orange and unsweetened iced tea instead of orange juice
Low-calorie vinaigrette instead of blue cheese salad dressing
Butter spray instead of butter
Vodka and diet tonic instead of vodka and tonic
Total savings: approximately 200 calories per day.

Physical Activity Increase

I need to exercise in the morning and get it out of the way, otherwise I won't do it.

On Saturday and Tuesday mornings, I will walk on the hiking trail up by the park that's right by the gardening center, where I go anyway. It will be perfect.

I'm going to try to weave in an additional fifteen minutes per day during the week. This will be pretty easy. I shop once a week, so I'll use that parking-lot scenario. At work, I will use parking lot C, which will probably save me time because there are always spots there.

I'm also going to start mowing the lawn once a week instead of having my son do it. I love that stuff anyway.

Above, you are laying out the particulars of how, what, where, and when.

a. What will you eat? (Suggestion: Make a detailed list of all your known Calorie Bargains.)
b. When will you increase your physical activity? (For example, two

weekdays during lunch hour, one weekend morning.)
Where? At the gym or elsewhere?
What sort of physical activity? (Aerobics? walking? weight training?)

Obstacles, Slipups, or Potential Setbacks I May Encounter in Pursuing My Goal

(Eating Alarm Times, Unconscious Eating, or Diet Busters)

a. At family gatherings, when I tend to overeat and throw my diet out the window
b. Lunchtime at the office—I eat at a fast-food restaurant twice a week
c. Dinner out two evenings per week. The bread basket!
d. Chinese food. We bring it in every week. I love it, and I'm not giving it up
e. Late-night snacking. Right after dinner, I'm ready to sit in front of the TV and have a bag of potato chips or ice cream. It's one or the other. And I know that brushing my teeth to avoid this craving is not going to cut it!
f. If I think I had something bad, I start eating everything in sight.

Ways to Overcome These Obstacles, Slipups, or Potential Setbacks

a. Prior to family gatherings, I will decide to bring my own food or ask the host to prepare something special that is not high in calories
b. Before eating at the fast-food restaurant, I will Mentally Rehearse going in and ordering two grilled-chicken sandwiches, without mayonnaise, and no fries. This will be instead of the large burger, fries, and a soda I usually have
c. I will make sure that I ask the waitperson not to bring any bread to the table, no matter with whom I'm dining. If someone wants bread, the server can put it on that person's individual plate. And if I really want the bread, I will ask for just one piece

d. I have no problem having my dumplings steamed instead of fried, and I could do without the soup noodles—that's not a big deal

e. Again, I'm going to prepare for late-night cravings by thinking in advance. I will not have any junk foods around. I tried Edy's/Dryers Slow-Churned Grand Light and it's pretty amazing, so I can have that occasionally, but I'm not going to keep it in the house—that's being a Diet Hero. When I want it, I will go out and buy it in the supermarket. If they don't have it, I will have one backup flavor, or I will not have any at all. As far as the chips go, I will use popcorn, air popped or pan made with Pam spray. Every time I eat that popcorn, I feel like I've cheated, and it's only about sixty calories for two full cups—I love it. I will also try to make sure I have my Life Preservers handy. I actually laminated them and put them in my wallet—they really do keep me focused

f. I will Mentally Rehearse cheating, and what happens next. It will not be a license to overeat. Instead, I will reach for one of my Calorie Bargains (e.g., two pieces of forty-calorie toast with I Can't Believe It's Not Butter spray and a little Splenda and cinnamon or Fudgsicles, etc.), and not go crazy bingeing.

Excuses I Might Use to Pull Me from My Goals

a. I really do have a slow metabolism, and it's so difficult to pay attention to everything I eat

b. I get embarrassed asking the waitstaff not to bring the bread to the table

c. My husband orders the Chinese food, so sometimes I have no control—he wants the fried dumplings. Not only that, but he doesn't always finish them all and then they're there to tempt me

d. Sometimes that low-calorie ice cream is on sale, so I like to buy it in quantity, and then it's in the house and I start to eat it every night. That defeats the purpose of having low-calorie ice cream in the first place.

Excuse Busters

a. Yes, I may have a slow metabolism, but I realize that I can make my new eating adjustments automatic and keep the weight off

b. I will call the restaurant right before I leave home and ask them over the phone, since I have less of a problem asking over the phone than in person

c. I will make sure that I do the ordering, or, at the very least, we can order fried dumplings for my husband and steamed for me

d. I figured out the actual cost by going out and buying low-calorie ice cream at full price, including the gas for each time I have to go to the supermarket, and it turns out that for an entire year's worth of ice cream it's about $25. That's pretty inexpensive compared to what I've spent on dieting over the years.

Long-Term Rewards

a. Fit into a great-looking bathing suit

b. Reduce my chances of getting one or more of the seven serious diseases related to being overweight

c. Be happier and more self-aware

d. Increase self-confidence.

Life Preservers

a. Running into Cynthia [high school days teaser] at the grocery store

b. Not embarrassed at parent-teacher's conference

c. Going on a bike trip with my family.

That's the plan, in a nutshell. So, become your own architect and general contractor. Once you have a well-structured, working blueprint, you'll be able to refer to it whenever you're in doubt about how to proceed. It will become the basis for a good, sturdy, livable diet plan that's not going to blow over like a house of cards even when the environmental climate gets rough.

◀◀◀ EPILOGUE ▶▶▶

You've done it. You're on your way to *dieting no more*. I'm confident that after reading this book you are inspired, excited, and incredibly motivated, and have probably already started on the path toward creating an automatic and livable diet. I've no doubt that you now have every single tool and piece of information you need to break your fat patterns and lose weight—and keep it off—forever.

I'm gratified and energized to have been able to share with you what I've learned from my own experience, and the experiences of my many clients, and to provide you with convincing *evidence* from the best and the brightest scientists in the areas of diet, health, psychology, behavior modification, nutrition, and exercise. It's taken me decades of sifting, studying, selecting, and synthesizing to gather these tools, which you can use to create your Automatic Diet *right now*.

The process I've outlined is designed to help you become aware of your *negative* unconscious behaviors—basically making them conscious because that is the only way you can see them and fix them. Once you're aware, you can create and substitute newer, better patterns. Then those new patterns will become unconscious—automatic, even—so that you can live your life fitter, happier, and healthier.

If you follow this process you will succeed, not just because this book can somehow miraculously lose the weight *for* you, but because you will be armed with the knowledge and the power that will help you to change your life and achieve your goals for good.

◄◄◄ APPENDIX A ►►►
THE THREE-DAY FOOD CHALLENGE

If you've decided to accept my Three-Day Food Challenge, but have never kept a food diary and are not quite sure what to include and how to go about it, here are a few tips that will help to ensure that your diary includes all the information you'll need.

Remember, keep an eye out for:

▸ Eating Alarm Times: That time of day when you are most likely to overeat

▸ Unconscious Eating: Mindless eating

▸ Not being aware of the nutrition information of the food you consume

▸ Portion Distortion: You think the portions are small, but it's usually not the case. Portions are rarely what you think they are.

▸ Diet Buster Moments: An event (a fancy dinner, watching TV), situation, or even a certain food that triggers you to move away from your goals

▸ Emotional or Stress Eating: A mood (happiness, boredom, depression) that leads to eating

▸ Meal Patterns: Skipping meals or letting too much time lapse between meals usually leads to overeating later in the day

▸ Not Planning Ahead: If high calorie and high-fat foods appear frequently on your food diary in the form of fast-food meals or vending-machine snacks, it may be a sign of not planning ahead. A food diary allows you to see your weak spots and to plan for them

▸ Unbalanced Meals: Are some meals heavy on the carbs? Or maybe a protein overdose? Not choosing balanced meals can lead to excessive hunger, which in turn can result in overeating

▸ Too Many Calories: To put it simply, you may be taking in more calories than you're burning

Beware of Portion Distortion

As you now know, most people underestimate the size of the portions they're consuming, and if your diary is to be accurate, you really need to be as aware as possible of what you're actually eating. Your eyes may be deceiving you, especially if you're already desensitized to larger portions (as many Americans are). It would be useful to actually measure what you're eating from time to time—particularly if you're having trouble losing weight—but here are some useful equivalents you can refer to, particularly when you're on the go.

Bread, cereal, rice, and pasta	
½ cup of cooked cereal, rice, or pasta	A fist
1 cup of ready-to-eat cereal, popcorn, or crackers	Baseball
¼ cup of granola	Roll of scotch tape
Vegetables	
1 cup of raw leafy greens	Two handfuls
½ cup of other vegetables, cooked or chopped raw	A fist
Fruit	
One medium apple or orange	Tennis ball
½ cup of chopped, canned, or cooked fruit	Small fist
2 tablespoons of raisins	Ping-Pong ball

Milk, yogurt, and cheese	
1 cup of milk or yogurt	Hand holding tennis ball
1 ounce of cheese	Matchbox, one deli slice, your thumb
Meat, poultry, fish, beans, eggs, nuts	
3 ounces of cooked meat, fish, or poultry	Deck of cards, cassette tape
1 ounce of meat	Typical deli slice
1 teaspoon of butter or peanut butter	Your fingertip or a stamp
1 tablespoon of peanut butter	Your thumb
2 tablespoons of peanut butter	Ping-Pong ball
1 ounce of nuts	A handful or 10 to 12 pieces
Snacks	
1 ounce or 1 cup of chips, pretzels, nuts	A handful

Keep It Real

Just as important as being accurate about portion size is writing down all those sin foods—cake, candy, salty snacks, and other high-calorie, high-fat items—we sometimes seem to forget. Even something as seemingly innocuous as a few Hershey's Kisses or one Oreo cookie still adds up.

Write What You Feel

Food diaries are critical for identifying emotional eating behaviors. When you see on paper that you're eating ten cookies every time you feel anxious or stressed, you know you need to work on finding better outlets to handle your stress.

Keep Your Options Open

Create a few different ways to record what you're eating. Studies show that a small notebook that fits into your pocket or bag is the best way to keep you writing. Have extras on hand in the car, house, and office. Never give yourself the excuse that you didn't have a diary available to write down what you ate.

Create Your Own Food Diary

Here's a rundown of exactly what you should be recording.

Meal, Time, and Place

Record the approximate time you sit down to eat. This may help you find the eating schedule that works best for you. Also, record what meal it was (e.g., breakfast, mid-morning, etc.) and where you ate it (on the run, sitting at your desk, at a restaurant, etc.).

Hunger Level

Record your level of hunger on a scale of one to five, one being the least hungry and five being the most hungry. You should aim to be between three and four when you're eating. You never want to let yourself get too hungry, and you certainly don't want to eat when you're not hungry at all.

Dining Companions

Write down with whom you ate and what you talked about. This information could offer clues to Unconscious Eating or Stress Eating.

Feelings and Mood

Record how you feel before, during, and/or after you eat. Before is probably the most important because it can have the greatest effect on how and what you eat. Try to keep track of whether you have general feelings like being happy or sad, or specific ones like "stressed at work," "angry at spouse," or "having a great day." You will see that this really helps you pinpoint which emotions affect your eating habits the most.

Food and Drink

Record all the individual foods you eat and beverages you drink, including accurate portion sizes. Anything that goes into your mouth should be in your food diary—including drinks, little nibbles from the refrigerator, and bites from other people's plates!

Nutrient Information

Record the calories, fat, carbs, and protein for each food/meal you eat. Total your calories at the end of the day to make sure you are staying within your goal. You can do this while you're at home, while relaxing. There are several sources to get nutrient information, but a good place to start is the United States Department of Agriculture (USDA). They have a free database available on their Web site (http://www.nal.usda.gov/fnic/cgi-bin/nut_search.pl). Or, if you prefer, you can purchase any one of the many paperback books on the market that list the nutrient content of thousands of foods.

At the end of three days, your diary should provide you with a clear picture of what, how, when, and why you eat what you do.

MORE CALORIE BARGAINS

Glenny's Soy Crisps (Barbecue)

One bag (1.3 oz): 140 calories, 3 g fat, 18 g carbs

I've received a number of e-mails from clients recommending these crisps, and my family and friends swear by them. In fact, most people who eat them regularly are a bit fanatical. I was reluctant to try them at first. I thought, "Soy—how good could they taste?" But when I finally broke down and had some, I was impressed. They really are an excellent snack, especially if you're in a chips mood. You can eat an entire bag without guilt—the company actually calls it their "portion control" bag.

Healthy Choice Caramel Swirl Ice-Cream Sandwich

One sandwich (4 oz): 140 calories, 3 g fat, 27 g carbs

I've recommended this ice-cream sandwich to about thirty people, and every one of them (except one British friend who said she "doesn't like things with cookie bits") loved it. Yes, it's on the higher end when it comes to carbohydrates, but it's also portion controlled. When I have pints of ice cream in the freezer, it's just too easy to grab another spoonful every now and then. These individually wrapped treats make it much easier to have "just one." If you want ice cream (and not nonfat frozen yogurt or soy) and you're watching your calories, this is a good bet. The bad news is that they're not available in every supermarket, but the people from Healthy Choice assured me that "very soon" they will be readily available in a "grocery store near you."

La Tortilla Factory Whole-Wheat, Low-Carb/Low-Fat Tortillas (Garlic and Herb)

One tortilla (36 g): 50 calories, 2 g fat, 11 g carbs

A number of West Coast readers to my column e-mailed to report how great these can be for dieters and—lo and behold—they are. The good news is that they're low in carbs and have no trans fat, added sugar, or saturated fat. They also contain soy flour and are very high in fiber (8 g). You can enjoy them with eggs in the morning (instead of toast) or use them to make low-calorie pizza (spread with low-calorie tomato sauce and sprinkled with part-skim mozzarella). In fact, the possibilities are endless.

Cheerios

2 cups: 220 calories, 4 g fat, 44 g carbs

A one-half cup of skim milk adds 43 calories, 0 grams of fat, and 6 grams of carbohydrates. You can eat 2 cups and for only 220 calories. And to tell you the truth, I never eat Cheerios for breakfast—typically I have a bowl as a mid-afternoon snack when I'm starving. They are also great because they have a decent amount of fiber, so you feel full. Plus, they are packed with essential vitamins and minerals and were one of the first cereals to be certified by the American Heart Association for heart-protective benefits, including lowering cholesterol. I've worked around plenty of registered dietitians, and I always see them snacking on dry Cheerios. Don't laugh until you try it—either plain or with a bit of artificial sweetener, they're pretty tasty. Or you can try Honey-Nut and Multi-Grain, which have 120 calories per cup—the choice is yours.

Egg White Omelets with Vegetables

*Eight egg whites, ½ cup frozen spinach, ½ a medium green or red bell
pepper, and ½ cup mushrooms (coat the pan with a cooking spray):
176 calories, 0 g fat, 11 g carbs*

You will not be hungry after eating this huge omelet—that's if you
can even eat the entire thing. This is a real meal. It fills you up, it's
packed with protein, it can be made in a matter of minutes, and it's perfect for anyone who wants to stay in shape. Also, did you know you can
microwave eggs? Just combine the egg whites and vegetables in a bowl,
pop them into the microwave, and cook through (times vary). And if
you think egg whites won't taste like eggs, you're wrong. They taste
every bit as good as whole eggs, without any fat.

Fudgsicle (No Sugar Added)

One bar: 45 calories, 0.5 g fat, 8.5 g carbs

My father just loves these. He's a diabetic, and he feels that he's not
missing a thing when he has one of these treats. They are preportioned
(because they're on a stick), and they offer great, satisfying flavor.

Vlasic Dill Pickles

*The entire 24-ounce jar of dill pickle spears: 70 calories
(yes, for the entire jar), 0 g fat, 14 g carbs*

You can eat the entire jar of delicious pickle spears for just seventy
calories—but if you do that, be aware of the fact that you'll also be consuming *a lot* of sodium. Realistically, I don't see anyone eating an entire
jar, but even a few pickles taste great, make an easy snack, their crunch
can be especially satisfying when you're craving chips with a sandwich,
and they have almost no calories. Try keeping a jar in the fridge—serve
them with meals, or just have them on hand for those late-night refrigerator raids—they're certainly better than a fistful of cookies or a slice
of cake!

Progresso 99% Fat-Free Roasted Chicken with Wild Rice Soup

2½ cups (one can): 225 calories, 3.75 g fat, 30 g carbs

Eating this soup doesn't make you feel shortchanged. It's rich, filling, and tasty, with lots of roasted, white-meat chicken. Eating a nice bowl of soup fills you up and psychologically makes you feel as if you've eaten a real meal.

Edy's (Dreyer's) Grand Light French Silk Ice Cream

1 cup (let's be realistic): 260 calories, 9 g fat (unfortunately it does contain trans fats—partially hydrogenated coconut oil), 38 g carbs

They have a "slow-churn" process so it maintains a great flavor, and it tastes great.

Sugar-Free Jell-O with Added Fruit (All Flavors)

The nutrition information below is the total amount for two entire packages, all eight servings—so if you want to, you can really stuff yourself and still not pack on the pounds.

Sugar-Free Jell-O: *(Serving size: 4 cups) 80 calories, 0 g fat, 0 g carbs*

    With ½ banana: *63 calories, 0 g fat, 16 g carbs*

    With ⅔ cup blueberries: *54 calories, 0 g fat, 14 g of carbs*

    Total for the entire batch: *197 calories, 0 g fat, 30 g carbs*

(Yes, that's it for all that Jell-O.)

◄◄◄ REFERENCES ►►►

Ackerman CJ, Turkoski B. (2000). "Using guided imagery to reduce pain and anxiety." *Home Health Nurse* 18(8):524–30; quiz 531.

Alfenas RC, Mattes RD. (2003). "Effect of fat sources on satiety." *Obesity Research* 11(2):183–7.

The American Institute for Cancer Research (2003). Awareness and Action: AICR Surveys on Portion Size, Nutrition, and Cancer Risk. Accessed on February 10, 2004, at http://www.aicr.org/press/awarenessandaction_03conf.pdf.

Andersen R, Wadden T, Bartlett S, Zemel B, Verde T, Franckowiak S. (1999). "Effects of lifestyle activity vs. structured aerobic exercise in obese women: a randomized trial." *Journal of the American Medical Association* 281:335–340

Anderson JW, Konz EC, Frederich RC, Wood CL. (2001). "Long-term weight-loss maintenance: a meta-analysis of US studies." *American Journal of Clinical Nutrition* 74(5):579–84.

———, Vichitbandra S, Qian W, Kryscio RJ. (1999). "Long-term weight maintenance after an intensive weight-loss program." *Journal of the American College of Nutrition* 18(6):620–7.

Bar-Eli M, Tenenbaum G, Pie JS, Btesh Y, Almog A. (1997). "Effect of goal difficulty, goal specificity and duration of practice time intervals on muscular endurance performance." *Journal of Sports Science* 15(2):125–35.

Barkeling B, Linne Y, Melin E, Rooth P. (2003). "Vision and eating behavior in obese subjects." *Obesity Research* 11(1):130–4.

Bell EA, Thorwart ML, Rolls BJ. (1998). "Effects of energy content and volume on sensory-specific satiety." *FASEB Journal,* b;12:A347(abs.).

Berry MW, Danish SJ, Rinke WJ, Smiciklas-Wright H. (1989). "Work-site health promotion: the effects of a goal-setting program on nutrition-related behaviors." *Journal of the American Dietetic Association* 89(7):914–20, 923.

Blackburn GL, MD, PhD. "Weight Management Expert Column Making Scientific Sense of Different Dietary Approaches. Part 2: Evaluating the Diets Posted 03/09/2004 Introduction and Dietary Approaches, Medscape Diabetes & Endocrinology." Accessed on March 19, 2004, at http://www.med scape.com/viewarticle/470747.

Brown JL, Miller D. (2002). "Couples' gender role preferences and management of family food preferences." *Journal of Nutrition Education and Behavior* 34(4):215–23.

Brownson RC, Chang JJ, Eyler AA, Ainsworth BE, Kirtland KA, Saelens BE, Sallis JF. (2004). "Measuring the environment for friendliness toward physical activity: a comparison of the reliability of 3 questionnaires." *American Journal of Public Health* 94(3):473–483.

Byrne SM. (2002). "Psychological aspects of weight maintenance and relapse in obesity." *Journal of Psychosomatic Research* 53(5):1029–36. Review.

Centers for Disease Control and Prevention. (2004). "Citing 'Dangerous Increase' in Deaths, HHS Launches New Strategies Against Overweight Epidemic." US Department of Health & Human Services. Accessed on March 9, 2004, at http://www.hhs.gov/news/press/2004pres/20040309.html.

Chandon P, Wansinki B. (2002). "Does stockpiling accelerate consumption? A convenience-salience framework of consumption." *Journal of Marketing Research* 39(3): 321–335.

Cho S, Dietrich M, Brown CJ, Clark CA, Block G. (2003). "The effect of breakfast type on total daily energy intake and body mass index: results from the Third National Health and Nutrition Examination Survey (NHANES III)." *Journal of the American College of Nutrition* 22(4):296–302.

Collet C, Roure R, Delhomme G, Dittmar A, Rada H, Vernet-Maury E. (1999). "Autonomic nervous system responses as performance indicators among volleyball players." *European Journal of Applied Physiology and Occupational Physiology* 80(1):41–51.

Conn VS. (1998). "Older adults and exercise: path analysis of self-efficacy related constructs." *Nursing Research* 47(3):180–9.

Cousins SO. (2003). "A self-referent thinking model: how older adults may talk themselves out of being physically active." *Health Promotion Practice* 4(4):439–48.

Dallow CB, Anderson J. (2003). "Using self-efficacy and a transtheoretical model to develop a physical activity intervention for obese women." *American Journal of Health Promotion* 17(6):373–81.

DiMeglio DP, Mattes RD. (2000). "Liquid versus solid carbohydrate: effects on food intake and body weight." *International Journal of Obesity and Related Metabolic Disorders* 24(6):794–800.

Dishman RK. (1994). "Motivating older adults to exercise." *Southern Medical Journal* 87(5):S79–82.

Drewnowski A. (1998). "Energy density, palatability, and satiety: implications for weight control." *Nutrition Reviews* 56:347–353.

———. (1997). "Taste preferences and food intake." *Annual Review of Nutrition* 17:237–53. Review.

Easterbrook G. "All This Progress Is Killing Us, Bite by Bite," *New York Times*, March 14, 2004, p. 5.

Epstein R. (May 1999). "Helping Athletes Go for the Gold," *Psychology Today*. Accessed at http://www.psychologytoday.com/htdocs/prod/ptoarticle/pto-19990501-000018.asp.

Ewing R, Schmid T, Killingsworth R, Zlot A, Raudenbush S. (2003). "Relationship between urban sprawl and physical activity, obesity, and morbidity." *American Journal of Health Promotion* 18(1):47–57.

Eyler AA, Baker E, Cromer L, King AC, Brownson RC, Donatelle RJ. (1998). "Physical activity and minority women: a qualitative study." *Health Education & Behavior* 25(5):640–52.

———, Brownson RC, Bacak SJ, Housemann RA. (2003). "The epidemiology of walking for physical activity in the United States." *Medicine and Science in Sports and Exercise* 35(9):1529–36.

Flatt JP. (1988). "Importance of nutrient balance in body-weight regulation." *Diabetes/Metabolism Review* 4(6):571–81. Review.

Fletcher, AM. *Eating Thin for Life: Food Secrets & Recipes from People Who Have Lost Weight & Kept It Off.* Boston: Houghton Mifflin Company, 1997.

———. *Thin for Life: 10 Keys to Success from People Who Have Lost the Weight & Kept It Off.* Boston: Houghton Mifflin Company, 2003.

Foster GD, Wadden TA, Vogt RA, Brewer G. (1997). "What is a reasonable weight loss? Patients' expectations and evaluations of obesity treatment outcomes." *Journal of Consulting and Clinical Psychology* 65(1):79–85.

French SA, Harnack L, Jeffery RW. (2000). "Fast-food restaurant use among women in the Pound of Prevention study: dietary, behavioral and demographic correlates." *International Journal of Obesity and Related Metabolic Disorders* 24(10):1353–9.

Frith M. (2003). "The unpalatable truth about the Atkins diet: it's just fatheaded nonsense, claim scientists," *The Independent*, August 13. Accessed on March 7, 2004 on the Internet at http://news.independent.co.uk/uk/health/story.jsp?story=433139.

Fussman C. (August 1998). "Jack Be Nimble, Jack Be Quick, Jack Saved My Fat Ass," *Esquire*, pp. 128–30.

General Mills Consumer Research Services Convenience Study. (2001). Author conducted interview with Heidi Geller Brand Public Relations via e-mail dated Monday, March 8, 2004.

Golan M, Crow S. (2004). "Parents are key players in the prevention and treatment of weight-related problems." *Nutrition Reviews* 62(1):39–50.

Hays NP, Starling RD, Liu X, Sullivan DH, Trappe TA, Fluckey JD, Evans WJ. (2004). "Effects of an ad libitum low-fat, high-carbohydrate diet on body weight, body composition, and fat distribution in older men and women: a randomized controlled trial." *Archives of Internal Medicine* 26;164(2):210–7.

Hall JC. (2002). "Imagery practice and the development of surgical skills." *American Journal of Surgery* 184(5):465–70. Review.

Hannum SM, Carson L, Evans EM, Canene KA, Petr EL, Bui L, Erdman JW Jr. (2004). "Use of portion-controlled entrees enhances weight loss in women." *Obesity Research* 12(3):538–46.

Hetherington MM. (1996). "Sensory-specific satiety and its importance in meal termination." *Neuroscience and Biobehavioral Reviews* 20(1):113–7.

Hill JO, Wyatt HR, Reed GW, Peters JC. (2003). "Obesity and the environment: where do we go from here?" *Science* 7;299(5608):853–5.

Hoch, SJ, Bradlow EL, Wansink B. (1999). "The variety of assortment." *Marketing Science* 18(4):527–46.

Hobden K, Pliner P. (1995). "Effects of a model on food neophobia in humans." *Appetite* 25(2):101–13.

Horovitz B. "You Want It Your Way." *USA Today*, March 5, 2004, p. A.1.

Jakicic JM. (2002). "The role of physical activity in prevention and treatment of body weight gain in adults." *Journal of Nutrition* 132(12):3826S–9S.

———. (2003). "Exercise in the treatment of obesity." *Endocrinology and Metabolism Clinics of North America* 32(4):967–80. Review.

———, Marcus BH, Gallagher KI, Napolitano M, Lang W. (2003). "Effect of exercise duration and intensity on weight loss in overweight, sedentary women: a randomized trial." *Journal of the American Medical Association* 290 (10):1323–30.

———, Wing RR, Butler BA, Robertson RJ. (1995). "Prescribing exercise in multiple short bouts versus one continuous bout." *International Journal of Obesity and Related Metabolic Disorders* 19:893–901.

———, Winters C, Lang W, Wing RR. (1999). "Effects of intermittent exercise and use of home exercise equipment on adherence, weight loss, and fitness in overweight women: a randomized trial." *Journal of the American Medical Association* 282:1554–60.

Jeffery RW, Rick AM. (2002). "Cross-sectional and longitudinal associations between body mass index and marriage-related factors." *Obesity Research* 10(8): 809–15.

Johnson SH. (2000). "Thinking ahead: the case for motor imagery in prospective judgments of prehension." *Cognition* 10;74(1):33–70.

Jones G, Cale A. (1997). "Goal difficulty, anxiety and performance." *Ergonomics* 40(3):319–33.

Kiernan M, King AC, Kraemer HC, Stefanick ML, Killen JD. (1998). "Characteristics of successful and unsuccessful dieters: an application of signal detection methodology." *Annals of Behavioral Medicine* 20, 1–6.

King AC, Castro C, Wilcox S, Eyler AA, Sallis JF, Brownson RC. (2000). "Personal and environmental factors associated with physical inactivity among different racial-ethnic groups of US middle-aged and older-aged women." *Health Psychology* 19(4):354–64.

Klem ML, Wing RR, Lang W, McGuire MT, Hill JO. (2000). "Does weight loss maintenance become easier over time?" *Obesity Research* 8(6):438–44.

———, Wing RR, McGuire MT, Seagle HM, Hill JO. (1997). "A descriptive study of individuals successful at long-term maintenance of substantial weight loss." *American Journal of Clinical Nutrition* 66(2):239–46.

Kristensen ST, Holm L, Raben A, Astrup A. (2002). "Achieving 'proper' satiety in different social contexts—qualitative interpretations from a cross-disciplinary project, sociomæt." *Appetite* 39(3):207–15.

Laitakari J, Vuori I, Oja P. (1996). "Is long-term maintenance of health-related physical activity possible? An analysis of concepts and evidence." *Health Education Research* 11(4):463–77. Review.

Laura Wilkinson Athlete Bio. http://www.usoc.org/cfdocs/athlete_bios/bio_template.cfm?ID=361&Sport=Diving 3/20/2004.

Levy D. "Athletes Learn to Train Their Minds, Too." *USA Today*, July 17, 1996, p. 05.D.

Lichtman SW, Pisarska K, Berman ER, Pestone M, Dowling H, Offenbacher E, Liebman B. (January/February 2004). "Weighing the diet books." *Nutrition Action* 31(1) 1, 3–5.

Liebman, B. (March 2004). "Food illusions." *Nutrition Action* 31(2):1, 3–6.

Locke EA, Latham GP. (2002). "Building a practically useful theory of goal setting and task motivation: A 35-year odyssey." *American Psychologist* 57(9): 705–17.

Lowe MR. (2003). "Self-regulation of energy intake in the prevention and treatment of obesity: is it feasible?" *Obesity Research* 11 Suppl:44S–59S. Review.

Ludwig DS. (2002). "The glycemic index: physiological mechanisms relating to obesity, diabetes, and cardiovascular disease." *Journal of the American Medical Association* 8;287(18):2414–23. Review.

Ma Y, Bertone ER, Stanek EJ III, Reed GW, Hebert JR, Cohen NL, Merriam PA, Ockene IS. (2003). "Association between eating patterns and obesity in a free-living US adult population." *American Journal of Epidemiology* 1;158(1): 85–92.

Martins Y, Pelchat ML, Pliner P. (1997). " 'Try it; it's good and it's good for you': Effects of taste and nutrition information on willingness to try novel foods." *Appetite* 28(2):89–102.

Mattes RD. (2002). "Feeding behaviors and weight loss outcomes over 64 months." *Eating Behaviors* 3(2):191–204.

———. (2002). "Ready-to-eat cereal used as a meal replacement promotes weight loss in humans." *Journal of the American College of Nutrition* 21(6):570–7.

McCrory MA, Fuss PJ, McCallum JE, Yao M, Vinken AG, Hays NP, Roberts SB. (1999). "Dietary variety within food groups: association with energy intake and body fatness in men and women." *American Journal of Clinical Nutrition* 69(3):440–7.

———, Fuss PJ, Saltzman E, Roberts SB. (2000). "Dietary determinants of energy intake and weight regulation in healthy adults." *Journal of Nutrition* 130(2S Suppl):276S–279S. Review.

———, Suen VM, Roberts SB. (2002). "Biobehavioral influences on energy intake and adult weight gain." *Journal of Nutrition* 132(12):3830S–4S.

McGuire MT, Wing RR, Klem ML, Hill JO. (1999). "Behavioral strategies of individuals who have maintained long-term weight losses." *Obesity Research* 7(4):334–41.

———, Wing RR, Klem ML, Lang W, Hill JO. (1999). "What predicts weight regain in a group of successful weight losers?" *Journal of Consulting and Clinical Psychology* 67(2):177–85.

————, Wing RR, Klem ML, Seagle HM, Hill JO. (1998). "Long-term mainte-nance of weight loss: do people who lose weight through various weight loss methods use different behaviors to maintain their weight?" *International Journal of Obesity and Related Metabolic Disorders* 22(6):572–7.

Metz JA, Stern JS, Kris-Etherton P, Reusser ME, Morris CD, Hatton DC, Oparil S, Haynes RB, Resnick LM, Pi-Sunyer FX, Clark S, Chester L, McMahon M, Snyder GW, McCarron DA. (2000). "A randomized trial of improved weight loss with a prepared meal plan in overweight and obese patients: impact on cardiovascular risk reduction." *Archives of Internal Medicine* 24;160(14):2150–8.

Millard M, Mahoney C, Wardrop J. (2001). "A preliminary study of mental and physical practice on the kayak wet exit skill." *Perceptual and Motor Skills* 92(3 Pt 2):977–84.

National Institutes of Health, National Heart Lung and Blood Institute. (1998). "Clinical guidelines on the identification, evaluation, and treatment of overweight and obesity in adults: the evidence report." *Obesity Research* 6(suppl. 2). Accessed at http://www.nhlbi.nih.gov/guidelines/obesity/prctgd_c.pdf.

Nielsen SJ, Popkin BBM. (2003). "Patterns of food portion sizes, 1997–1998." *Journal of the American Medical Association* 289:450–3.

Novotny JA, Rumpler WV, Judd JT, Riddick PH, Rhodes D, McDowell M, Briefel R. (2001). "Diet interviews of subject pairs: how different persons re-call eating the same foods." *Journal of the American Dietetic Association* 101(10):1189–93.

————, Rumpler WV, Riddick H, Hebert JR, Rhodes D, Judd JT, Baer DJ, Mc-Dowell M, Briefel R. (2003). "Personality characteristics as predictors of un-derreporting of energy intake on 24-hour dietary recall interviews." *Journal of the American Dietetic Association* 103(9):1146–51.

Ogden J. (2000). "The correlates of long-term weight loss: a group compari-son study of obesity." *International Journal of Obesity and Related Metabolic Disor-ders* 24(8):1018–25.

Orlick T, Partington J. (1988). "Mental links to excellence." *Sport Psychologist* 2(2):105–30.

Painter E, Wansink B, Hieggelke JB. (2002). "How visibility and convenience influence candy consumption." *Appetite* 38(3):237–8.

Paivio A. (1985). "Cognitive and motivational functions of imagery in human performance." *Canadian Journal of Applied Sport Sciences* 10(4):22S–28S.

Pontari BA, Schlenker BR, Christopher AN. (2002). "Excuses and character: Identifying the problematic aspects of excuses." *Journal of Social and Clinical Psychology* 21: 497–516.

Rauschenbach B, Sobal J, Frongillo EA Jr. (1995). "The influence of change in marital status on weight change over one year." *Obesity Research* 3: 319–27.

Richards D. (1985). "A perspective for visionaries." *Journal for Quality and Participation* 20–24.

Roach JB, Yadrick MK, Johnson JT, Boudreaux LJ, Forsythe WA III, Billon W. (2003). "Using self-efficacy to predict weight loss among young adults." *Journal of the American Dietetic Association* 103(10):1357–9.

Rolls BJ, Bell EA. (1999). "Intake of fat and carbohydrate: role of energy density." *European Journal of Clinical Nutrition* 53 (Suppl. 1):S166–73.

———. (2000). "The role of energy density in the overconsumption of fat." *The Journal of Nutrition* 130(2S Suppl.):268S–71S. Review.

———. (2002). *The Volumetrics Weight-Control Plan: Feel Full on Fewer Calories.* New York: HarperTorch, 2002.

Roure R, Collet C, Deschaumes-Molinaro C, Delhomme G, Dittmar A, Vernet-Maury E. (1999). "Imagery quality estimated by autonomic response is correlated to sporting performance enhancement." *Integrative Physiological and Behavioral Science* 66(1):63–72.

Schlenker BR. (1997). "Personal responsibility: Applications of the triangle model." In L.L. Cummings & B. Staw (eds.), *Research in Organizational Behavior* (Vol. 19, pp. 241–301). Greenwich, CT: JAI.

———, Pontari BA, Christopher AN (2001). "Excuses and character: Personal and social implication of excuses." *Personality and Social Psychology Review* 5:15–32.

Schlosberg S. (August 1998). "Let's Get Visual: With the Right Techniques, Weight Training Success Is All in Your Head." *Men's Fitness.* Accessed at http://articles.findarticles.com/p/articles/mi_m1608/is_n8_v14/ai_210320 39/print.

Serdula MK, Mokdad AH, Williamson DF, Galuska DA, Mendlein JM, Heath GW. (1999). "Prevalence of attempting weight loss and strategies for controlling weight." *Journal of the American Medical Association* 282:1353–8.

Sherwood NE, Jeffery RW, French SA, Hannan PJ, Murray DM. (2000). "Predictors of weight gain in the Pound of Prevention study." *International Journal of Obesity* 24:395–403.

Shick SM, Wing RR, Klem ML, McGuire MT, Hill JO, Seagle H. (1998). "Persons successful at long-term weight loss and maintenance continue to consume a low-energy, low-fat diet." *Journal of the American Dietetic Association* 98(4):408–13.

Shide DJ, Rolls BJ. (1995). "Information about the fat content of preloads influences energy intake in healthy women." *Journal of the American Dietetic Association* 95(9):993–8.

Sifton, Sam. "What He Ate: A Food Diary from New York." *New York Times,* March 31, 2004, p. D1.

Slentz CA, Duscha BD, Johnson JL, Ketchum K, Aiken LB, Samsa GP, Houmard JA, Bales CW, Kraus WE. (2004). "Effects of the amount of exercise on body weight, body composition, and measures of central obesity: STRRIDE—A randomized controlled study." *Archives of Internal Medicine* 164: 31–39.

Smicklas-Wright H, Mitchell DC, Mickle SJ, Goldman JD, Cook A. (2003). "Foods commonly eaten in the United States, 1989–1991; are portion sizes changing?" *Journal of the American Dietetic Association* 103:41–47.

Sobal J, Rauschenbach B, Frongillo EA. (2003). "Marital status changes and body weight changes: a US longitudinal analysis." *Social Science & Medicine* 56(7):1543–55.

Stallberg-White C, Pliner P. (1999). "The effect of flavor principles on willingness to taste novel foods." *Appetite* 33(2):209–21.

Stephens R. (1993). "Imagery: a strategic intervention to empower clients. Part I—Review of research literature." *Clinical Nurse Specialist* 7(4):170–4. Review.

Stirling LJ, Yeomans MR. (2004). "Effect of exposure to a forbidden food on eating in restrained and unrestrained women." *International Journal of Eating Disorders* 35(1):59–68.

Stone WJ, Klein DA. (March/April 2004). "Long-term exercisers: what can we learn from them?" *ACSM Health & Fitness Journal* (8)2:11–13.

Stutts WC. (2002). "Physical activity determinants in adults. Perceived benefits, barriers, and self efficacy." *Official Journal of the American Association of Occupational Health Nurses* 50(11):499–507.

Taylor JA, Shaw DF. (2002). "The effects of outcome imagery on golf-putting performance." *Journal of Sports Sciences* 20(8):607–13.

Taylor SE, Pham LB, Rivkin ID, Armor DA. (1998). "Harnessing the imagination. Mental simulation, self-regulation, and coping." *American Psychologist* 53(4):429–39.

Theodorakis Y, Laparidis K, Kioumourtzoglou E, Goudas M. (1998). "Combined effects of goal setting and performance feedback on performance and physiological response on a maximum effort task." *Perceptual and Motor Skills* 86(3 Pt 1):1035–41.

"The Truth About Dieting." (June 2002). *Consumer Reports* 67:25–31.

"Too Little Exercise, Rather Than Eating Too Much, Seen as Biggest Cause of Obesity." *The Wall Street Journal.* Poll conducted by Harris Poll (R) of Harris Interactive. Vol. 3, Issue 7, April 6, 2004, online. Accessed on April 6, 2004 at http://www.harrisinteractive.com/news/newsletters_wsj.asp.

Wansink, B. (December 1994). "Antecedents and mediators of eating bouts." *Family and Consumer Sciences Research Journal* 23(2):166–82.

———. (1993). "Bet you can't eat just one: what stimulates consumption acceleration?" *Journal of Food Products Marketing* 1(4):1–26.

———. "Bottoms Up! Peripheral Cues and Consumption Volume." *Food Psychology.* Accessed on February 17, 2004, at http://www.foodpsychology.com/overeating.html.

———. (1996). "Can package size accelerate usage volume?" *Journal of Marketing* 60(3):1–14.

———. (2002). "Changing eating habits on the home front: lost lessons from World War II research." *Journal of Public Policy & Marketing* 21(1):90–9.

———, Linder LR. (2003). "Interactions between forms of fat consumption and restaurant bread consumption." *International Journal of Obesity and Related Metabolic Disorders* 27(7):866–8.

———, Rohit D. (January 1994). "'Out of sight, out of mind': the impact of household stockpiling on usage rates." *Marketing Letters* 5(1):91–100.

———, Sangerman C. (2000). "Engineering comfort foods." *American Demographics* 22(7):66–7.

———, SeaBum P. (2001). "At the movies: how external cues and perceived tastes impact consumption." *Food Quality and Preference Journal* 12(1):69–74.

Weisel H, Heshka S, Matthews DE, Heymsfield SB. (1992). "Discrepancy between self-reported and actual caloric intake and exercise in obese subjects." *New England Journal of Medicine* 327(27):1893–8.

Weng HH, Bastian LA, Taylor DH Jr, Moser BK, Ostbye T. (2004). "Number of children associated with obesity in middle-aged women and men: results from the health and retirement study." *Journal of Women's Health* 13(1):85–91.

Westerterp-Plantenga MS, Lejeune MP, Nijs I, van Ooijen M, Kovacs EM. (2004). "High protein intake sustains weight maintenance after body weight loss in humans." *International Journal of Obesity and Related Metabolic Disorders* 28(1):57–64.

Williams SP. "Losing Weight: It's All in the Snacks." *Newsweek,* March 25, 2002. Accessed at http://www.keepmedia.com/pubs/Newsweek/2002/03/25/310902.

"Why Americans Are Losing the Fat Fight." (2004). CNN.com, March 25, 2004. Accessed on March 31, 2004, at http://www.cnn.com/2004/HEALTH/03/25/obesity.conference.reut/index.html.

Wing RR, Hill JO. (2001). "Successful weight loss maintenance." *Annual Review of Nutrition* 21:323–41. Review.

Wurtman RJ, Wurtman JJ.(1995). "Brain serotonin, carbohydrate-craving, obesity and depression." *Obesity Research* 3:477S–80S.

Wyatt HR, Grunwald GK, Mosca CL, Klem ML, Wing RR, Hill JO. (2002). "Long-term weight loss and breakfast in subjects in the National Weight Control Registry." *Obesity Research* 10(2):78–82.

◄◄◄ INDEX ►►►

◄◄◄ ABOUT THE AUTHOR ►►►

Charles Stuart Platkin is one of the country's leading nutrition and public-health advocates whose syndicated nutrition and fitness column appears in more than 155 daily newspapers nationally, including the *New York Post,* the *Miami Herald,* the *Seattle Times,* the *Orange County Register,* *Buffalo News,* and the *Richmond Times-Dispatch.* He is the founder and director of The Institute for Nutrition & Behavioral Sciences, a nonprofit organization that conducts obesity-related research and designs public-health programs. Platkin is also the founder of two companies— Integrated Wellness Solutions and Nutricise—that deliver weight control and health information and advice to individuals throughout the country. Integrated Wellness Solutions provides a sophisticated online software program that integrates cutting-edge scientific research and the latest in "behavioral nutrition" research. The program is used by insurance and pharmaceutical companies, fitness centers, and other large corporations to assist more than 500,000 people each year in losing weight and increasing their physical activity. Nutricise is the first program to offer individuals one-on-one weight-control counseling with registered dietitians via e-mail. The company has counseled more than 100,000 people, helping them to understand that choosing to lose weight is not simply about choosing what we put in our mouths, but about choosing how we live our lives.

Platkin has been quoted as a weight loss/nutrition expert in numerous publications, including *USA Today,* the *Los Angeles Times,* the *Chicago Tribune, Time, Newsweek, Ladies' Home Journal, Men's Health, Shape,* and

Fitness; he has also appeared on NBC's *The Today Show*, CNN, CNBC, CBS's *The Early Show*, the BBC, and others. He received his Masters in Public Health from Florida International University, and he is a member of the American Society for Nutritional Sciences, the American Obesity Association, the North American Association for the Study of Obesity, the National Strength and Conditioning Association, and the American Council on Exercise. He received a law degree from Fordham University, and his undergraduate degree from Cornell University. He is also a certified personal trainer.

His first book, *Breaking the Pattern* (www.breakingthepattern.com), was a self-help bestseller in hardcover; it has been used by addiction clinics to assist patients with resolving drug and alcohol–related issues and more than twenty universities around the country as a text to teach behavioral-change techniques to nutrition and dietetic counseling students.